After the Storm . . . There is the Calm

With much affection, I dedicate this book to Tamika and Aisha
who have shared a special part of my life
May they continue to be blessed

After the Storm . . . There is the Calm

An Analysis of the Bereavement Process

Audrey Pottinger

Canoe Press
University of the West Indies
Barbados • Jamaica • Trinidad and Tobago

Canoe Press University of the West Indies
1A Aqueduct Flats Mona
Kingston 7 Jamaica

© 1999 by Audrey M. Pottinger
All rights reserved. Published 1999
ISBN 13: 978-976-8125-50-7

03 02 01 00 99   5 4 3 2 1

CATALOGUING IN PUBLICATION DATA
Pottinger, Audrey M.
  After the storm . . . there is the calm / Audrey Pottinger M.

p. cm.
Includes bibliographical references and index.

1. Grief. 2. Bereavement – Psychological aspects.
3. Loss (Psychology). 4. Death – Psychological aspects.
I. Title.
BF724.3.G73P68 1999   155.937

The short story on pages 11 and 12 is reproduced with the permission of the writer, Nikola Nolan

CONTENTS

Foreword		vii
Preface		ix
Introduction		xiii
Chapter 1	Grieving: Phases and Symptoms	1
Chapter 2	Social and Psychological Effects of Loss	10
Chapter 3	Bereavement Outcomes	14
Chapter 4	Theoretical Explanations of Grief	20
Chapter 5	Bereavement in Childhood.	31
Chapter 6	Suicide	37
Chapter 7	Death by Murder and from AIDS	47
Chapter 8	Intervention	55
Appendix		65
Bibliography		82
Index		86

FOREWORD

When I was asked to write this foreword, I found it both threatening and challenging. Threatening because I was grieving a loss; challenging because of the possibilities for growth in the process of managing the consequences of loss. I am glad I responded positively to the request in the end.

I endorse this book as a work that offers much support and help in the storm of grieving. In the text Dr Pottinger takes this common and everyday subject and, with her wealth of knowledge, personal experience and contacts with grieving people, informs and guides those who suffer loss and those who seek to help them.

Although her own cultural experiences are clearly seen in some of the conclusions and interpretations she offers, *After the Storm . . . There Is the Calm* has universal appeal and application.

Her reflections on grieving children are timely. They tend to be overlooked when the subject is addressed. But as more and more they become the tragic victims of loss, Dr Pottinger speaks to all of us: "The importance of helping a child to accept and grieve cannot be overstated."

Suicide, AIDS and murder frighten us with their growing statistics and the closeness with which we face them almost daily. With her insight in dealing with human nature, we are helped to face, to bear, and to grow in dealing with the grief related to loss.

Finally, as Dr Pottinger draws attention to some mistakes commonly made by those who relate to grieving people, we are given some clues that can help us avoid unnecessary pain and embarrassment.

Pastors, counsellors, teachers, hospital personnel and the average human being have, in this text, much to think about as they seek to calm those who go through the storm of grieving.

J. Oliver Daley
Moderator, United Church of Jamaica and the Cayman Islands

PREFACE

Since my sojourn in the field of bereavement about a decade ago, I have met with individuals who have vehemently resisted my explanations of why I felt it necessary and worthwhile to specialize in working with the bereaved. Their responses have been that death is something that happens to everyone, it is natural and you cannot take away the pain. Therefore, what is the use of studying it?

After doing academic research with the recently bereaved and the pre-bereaved (those who were facing an impending loss), I became increasingly aware that my goal would not be to try and help the bereaved avoid the pain of grief, as this was unrealistic and most probably unhelpful. However, if I better understood the intrapersonal and interpersonal processes of bereavement, the normal and pathological courses that grief can take, and the different sources of emotional pain, I would be better equipped to help someone cope with the anxiety, fears and self-destructive behaviours that can accompany loss.

Thus, in spite of the existing taboo in speaking freely about death and dying, and despite the reactions from my friends, who refer to me as "the morbid one," I have ploughed on, giving lectures on the topic and working with the bereaved. I am sure that my writing a book on the subject has now sealed my fate as being "unduly interested in death."

This book is not a rule book on the right or wrong way to cope with a personal loss. It is a book of practical suggestions and advice that have been found to be helpful with the bereaved. It attempts to dispel some of the misperceptions about loss and bereavement. It addresses bereavement in children and differentiates it from the grief of adults. It presents bereavement in a theoretical and cultural framework for analysis. It provides information on those who are "at risk" for a poor adjustment and thus may need professional help. It looks at suicide in adults and adolescents and broadens our understanding of the suicide victim as well as the surviving family members. And it presents death by murder and AIDS as special losses that reflect the times and society in which the author lives.

I had delayed writing this book, since there are a number of books available on coping with bereavement. However, my travels and research experience have shown me that culture plays a significant role in shaping the bereavement process. Thus, although death is universal, man's experiences, coping skills and attitudes will vary depending on the cultural perspective from which he interprets the loss.

I am a Jamaican, a West Indian, who has lived in the Caribbean most of her life. I have studied and actively shared in the grief experiences of the bereaved from my culture as well as those of the bereaved from the USA and the UK. I have interviewed and counselled persons facing the impending death of a loved one from a terminal illness, as well as those who have recently been bereaved and those who have been bereaved for many years. I have worked in hospices and palliative care units and alongside health professionals who are dedicated to the field.

All of these experiences have certainly influenced my writing, but my interpretation of grief and loss has also been affected by my cultural upbringing. All of the known authors in this field are Europeans and North Americans. A book on bereavement written by a black West Indian therefore carries its own distinction. At the same time the information provided in this book should not be confining and ethnofocal because of my multicultural experiences. The research for this book was drawn mainly from North America, Scotland and Jamaica.

Many persons have supported my efforts at research and writing over the years. Prominent among them is my good friend and mentor, David A. Alexander. He initiated me in the field and guided me through years of study. I am very grateful to him. I am also indebted to my other colleagues who have studied the field far longer than I and have thus provided me with scientific evidence and anecdotal information to collate for my book. Their works are duly acknowledged throughout the book.

I would also like to acknowledge the support and encouragement of my family and friends, especially my sister and her husband, who provided me with comfort and a quiet place to complete the writing of this book.

The many bereaved individuals in Aberdeen, Kingston and Miami who willingly shared their experiences with me are also especially and sincerely thanked. It is my wish that this book will be a fitting testament to the pain and grief they endured and that the knowledge garnered will be useful in helping individuals survive grief.

This book is for anyone who is trying to cope with a loved one's death, or who finds himself in a position where he is called on to offer comfort to a friend who is grieving. It is also for the health professional and for the student who will be working with the bereaved. *After the Storm . . . There is the Calm is* based on my belief that each of us, when we are faced with a loss, has the capacity not just to cope with the loss, but to grow as a result of it.

Introduction

Most families can and do cope with bereavement without any professional intervention. However, over the past twenty years, health professionals have reported that referrals of psychological symptoms and physical complaints related to a loss are becoming more commonplace. Additionally, it is no longer atypical for individuals to seek the services of professionals while acutely grieving a recent loss. In my practice ten to fifteen percent of new clients receive bereavement counselling in any given year, and this number is likely to increase with the rising rates of homicide and suicide.

Many bereaved clients do not associate their present behaviours and concerns with their loss and therefore are unaware that they need grief counselling. One of my early cases was of a woman in her late thirties who had undergone exploratory surgery on her stomach three times. The doctors could find no physical cause for her symptoms. This woman's father had died of cancer of the stomach over a decade ago. After the third operation her general practitioner referred her for psychological counselling.

Other examples include the case of a young man in his early thirties, who had not practised setting any goals in his adult life because he believed he did not have a right to be happy. He had dropped out of college, had a history of short-lived relation-ships and marriages, and generally had poor interpersonal skills. In addition to other significant losses in his life, this man had witnessed the murder of his father when he was a teen.

A successful career woman in her thirties had a history of adulterous relationships. When she was ten her father, whom she had idolized, left the family home and she had not heard from him again.

The teacher of a child at preparatory school reported that the child had become disruptive in class since the beginning of the term, and that her grades had fallen. A classmate had died tragically earlier in the term. There was also the case of a nine year old boy who began sucking his finger in class, wetting his pants and clinging to his class teacher, shortly after his mother died.

There are also cases in which the clients or patients recognize the impact of the loss but are still unable to cope. A distraught husband sought help for his wife, who he felt was depressed and finding it difficult to function at work or relate to her family. His wife had recently experienced a miscarriage.

Some persons accept the death of a loved one intellectually, but years after the death are unable to speak about the deceased without breaking into tears, or are unable to look at a photograph or personal belongings of the deceased. These persons will voluntarily seek help when they feel they need to move on with their lives.

Grief and bereavement are examined at length in the following chapters. The book is organized to take its readers through defining and understanding grief, coping with loss and finding a healthy resolution. Traditionally, the bereavement response was classified as a depressive reaction or post-traumatic stress disorder. However, recently, there has been a trend among mental health workers to consider bereavement as having a distinct pattern and complications as well as specific treatment strategies. Chapter one opens with a description of uncomplicated grief, that is, the "normal" course that grief takes, and those symptoms that are typically experienced by the bereaved.

Some of the psychological and social effects of loss are dramatized in a short story in chapter two. Loss by divorce is the grief experience that is illustrated in this story. In this chapter the point is made graphically that bereavement is just one of many kinds of losses. The story is used to highlight the common bond that exists among major losses such as migration, divorce or death.

Chapter three illustrates how to diagnose pathological or complicated grief reactions, and also defines different types of bereavement outcomes. Chapter four examines three theoretical perspectives on coping with loss. These theories attempt to explain the different types of response to loss and also why some people cope better with a loss than others.

Many adults still have misunderstandings and misperceptions about a child's grief, believing it to be similar to the adult experience. However, there are distinct patterns of responses that are unique to a child's experience of loss. These are examined in chapter five. The child's grief response is interpreted and explained according to his or her age and cognitive level of functioning.

While I was writing this book, a family friend committed suicide. Because of my close attachment to the surviving family members I mourned with them and shared their grief and pain. I had not intended to include a chapter on suicide in this book, but because of this personal experience and the increased media attention to suicide in the USA and in Jamaica, I felt it could be helpful to take a closer look at this special kind of loss. Chapter six, therefore, focuses on the person at risk for suicide and the experience of family members and friends who are suicide survivors. In the latter part of this chapter, children and adolescent suicide victims are singled out as there is an alarming increase in the numbers of suicide in this age group.

A book on coping with bereavement, written by a Jamaican, would not be complete if a chapter was not dedicted to coping with death by murder, as well as death from AIDS. The former is, unfortunately, a common event in Jamaica which, with a population of 2.5 million, averaged more than two murders a day in 1996. AIDS is an epidemic worldwide and some of the characteristics of Jamaicans and Jamaica place its people at risk for this highly communicable disease (Figueroa et al. 1995). Jamaicans are mobile people with a long standing history of migratory patterns. They travel and work all over the world, while remaining in touch with their homeland. In addition, Jamaica is viewed by many as a mecca for tourists, and attracts hundred of thousands to its shores annually.

Death by murder and from AIDS have unique features which seem to complicate the grieving process for family members. They are presented as special losses, because coping with them does not seem to fit existing models on grief. The effect of these losses are just now being researched and documented. Chapter seven, therefore, should add to our understanding of them.

It can be argued that bereavement researchers, like myself, by attempting to explain normal and complicated forms of grief, are placing the right to decide how one should cope with a loss in the hands of a few professionals. Let me categorically state that there is no right or wrong way to respond to a loss. Bereavement researchers and workers recognize this and are not out to create "norms" of behaviours.

What research in this field has achieved is well documented information on effective intervention strategies. In addition to these interventions which are offered at the micro (individual) level, bereavement research has also affected public policy changes at the macro (societal) level. The development of hospice care services worldwide for the terminally ill and their relatives and the establishment of support groups for the bereaved are but two areas influenced by research. The inclusion of death education in the US school curriculum and its emphasis on preventative education is another tangible benefit of bereavement research.

In the final chapter of this book, I have identified social and demographic factors that heighten the need for professional intervention for the bereaved. Chapter eight also discusses intervention strategies for both bereaved adults and children. Practical suggestions are made for the bereaved themselves and guidance is offered for those who find themselves helping the bereaved. It is my intention to provide useful information and help to those who feel uncomfortable or helpless when faced with this subject.

CHAPTER 1

Grieving: Phases and Symptoms

What Is Grief Like?

It has been widely acknowledged that grieving a major loss occurs in clearly definable and predictable phases or stages. These stages can be observed in the individual who is confronted with a divorce, migration, loss of limb, failure of a major examination, or the death of a loved one. Knowledge of these phases can help to prepare the mourner or someone working with the bereaved about what to expect during mourning.

Phase One – Shock

A number of bereavement experts agree that the initial reaction to a significant loss is shock and denial (Kubler-Ross 1969; Raphael 1977; Murray Parkes 1970, 1972, 1986). The bereaved tend to report a sense of numbness or disbelief on hearing of the death of a significant other. This numbness can last for a few hours to weeks. The intensity and duration of the shock feeling depends on the circumstances of the loss and the support that is available from friends and family. Sudden, unexpected deaths are associated with a greater degree of shock and disbelief.

The disbelief seems to serve as a buffer, which permits the bereaved to gradually process the news of the loss. A bereaved friend once told me that it was as if God, who knows our mental strength, uses an initial denial period to protect us. She recalled the case of a secretary who heard about her husband's death at work. After she was called into her boss's office and informed of the death, she thanked him, excused herself, and went back to her desk and resumed typing. It was not until some hours later that she was able to absorb the news.

It is believed that how a person deals with the shock phase sets the trend for the course of grief. The bereaved who allow friends and relatives to help them through this initial period tend to continue to move with some ease through the different phases of grief. Individuals need the greatest physical support at this time because they are usually too stunned to think and make decisions. Neighbours who provide food, who come by and open windows in the house, and who are generally available to take care of the practical needs of the bereaved are offering the kind of support that is often needed at this time.

Shock tends to bring about feelings of helplessness. Thus, the bereaved in this vulnerable state can feel overwhelmed and develop strong feelings of dependency and insecurity. At times they will report that they do not want to be left alone. Whereas support is necessary and beneficial, requesting or seeking the company of others can help the bereaved to maintain feelings of denial, and to avoid dealing with the news of the loss.

In addition to the feelings of shock experienced during this first phase of grief, other commonly expressed feelings include confusion, restlessness, and alarm. The bereaved who are confused will comment that they feel that their world is being shattered and nothing will ever be the same again. These individuals tend to report that they find it difficult to think clearly and to make mundane decisions. They often begin fearing that they are "losing their minds".

Because of the confusion, some find comfort in movement. The ongoing activity prevents them from thinking about the loss. The bereaved who is restless may start doing a task and then leave it incomplete and begin to do something else. Health professionals offer a biological explanation for the restlessness experienced by some bereaved persons. They argue that because the body is in a state of shock or stress the sympathetic nervous system is geared for the "fight or flight" reaction. The body is thus on "alert", even if the person is exhausted.

The reactions during the initial phase of grieving are not confined to cognitive and psychological responses, but also include the physiological. When the body is in a state of shock its cardiovascular system can go into an alarm state, causing blood to be pumped away from the extremities, the hands and feet, to the head and trunk. This explains the icy fingers we sometimes observe in the recently bereaved.

Sweaty palms and trembling over the entire body are other signs related to the effects of adrenaline on various organs in the body. In addition, the body's immunity is lowered, thus making the bereaved more prone to contracting infections.

Phase Two – Processing the Loss

Although the bereaved may have started processing the loss shortly after receiving news of the death, the funeral tends to mark a psychological turning point for beginning the grieving process. The second phase of bereavement has begun. Friends, coworkers, peers, and family members who had clamoured around earlier leave shortly after and the bereaved person is left to mourn on his or her own and resume normal life. Contrary to popular perception, moving from an initial phase of grief, characterized by shock, into a stage of processing the loss is not an irreversible process. During this second phase the bereaved may still experience shock and periodically deny that the loss has occurred.

When left by themselves the bereaved begin to ruminate more frequently on the events leading to the death and the actual death event itself. They replay the visual images associated with the death in their minds and, by doing so, they gradually process the impact of the loss. It has been my experience that if the bereaved can recall the sequence of events clearly and not have their recall distorted, for example, by drugs to "deaden the pain", then this helps them in resolving the loss. It also appears to facilitate adjustment when the last image the bereaved has of the deceased is that of a body lying peacefully in a state of rest. When the image is gruesome and unpleasant, processing the loss appears to be more traumatic.

The bereaved often respond to the second phase of grief with intense anxiety accompanied by somatic complaints, such as loss of appetite, inability to sleep, dryness of the throat and mouth, and loss of energy. They, more or less, have accepted the death intellectually but may still be trying to assimilate the information emotionally. Accepting a loss is a slow and gradual process, characterized at times by raw pain. Anything can remind the bereaved of the deceased and the loss. Feelings and questions that were previously blocked will now emerge.

Persons who are experiencing normal and uncomplicated

grief report the need to cry, or they will appear sad-looking and depressed. They also commonly report feeling angry and guilty. These are all natural feelings. However, their intensity during a loss encounter and the simultaneous experience of a different number of emotions can create powerful feelings of inability to cope in the recently bereaved.

Crying

Crying is believed to be cathartic because, when we cry, it is as if our emotions are being discharged through our tears. However, there are times when the crying response is not available to the bereaved. When this happens over a prolonged period the inability to respond in this manner seems to exacerbate the bereaved's pain. I have heard people say, with pain in their voices, "I wish I could cry but I can't."

Feelings of sadness and the need to cry seem to occur in waves. At times bereaved persons will feel emotionally calm and 'tear-free' and other times they will report crying all night long. Accompanying the crying is a strong yearning for the deceased to return. Although intellectually the bereaved person knows this is impossible, the "child" inside wishes with all his or her heart that the deceased will return. The many "sightings" reported by family members of deceased loved ones seem to be testimony to this desire.

Anger

Anger is so commonly experienced by bereaved family members that its absence may be an indicator of complication in the grief process. Although the anger is expected, it is still considered one of the major sources of despair and discomfort in the bereaved. When a loved one dies there is the tendency to blame and this blaming forms the basis of what is experienced as anger.

Blame can be directed at many sources. Family and friends can be blamed for not being supportive at the time of the loss. Those who are directly or indirectly responsible for the death, either through murder or accident, can be blamed. The bereaved can blame medical doctors or God for not saving the life of the deceased. The deceased can also be blamed for contributing to their demise through careless living, or the bereaved may feel anger at the deceased for what they interpret as deserting them. There is also the act of self blame, when the bereaved blame themselves for negligent behaviour or for otherwise causing the death.

Blame resulting in anger is not always acknowledged or accepted by the bereaved and others. There are times when the bereaved will disguise, deny, suppress or repress their feelings because they feel it is inappropriate to express them. The bereaved may feel awkward at expressing negative feelings about the deceased because society expects them to only make positive statements at this time. Also, because of their need to protect the character of the deceased, the bereaved may deny their feelings of anger and resentment.

Many people will not admit to angry feelings when someone enquires directly. However, the bereaved person who tries hard not to express his or her anger tends to have nightmares and psychosomatic problems. On the other hand, the bereaved may act out their anger and be reckless, impulsive and destructive in their behaviours. Persons who do not constructively express their anger can also focus this anger inward and develop self destructive behaviours. These persons tend to be prone to depression and are often suicidal.

Guilt

Guilt is closely related to self blame and anger. It is experienced when surviving family members feel they could have done more for the deceased or done things differently. You will often hear a bereaved individual moaning "If only I had . . ." Some bereaved persons may also experience guilt as a result of their lack of expressions of feelings. They may believe that they are not experiencing, thus not expressing, the "appropriate amount" of sadness. In addition, when a parent loses a child, a sibling loses a brother or sister, and a spouse loses a partner, these persons may experience what has been termed "survivors' guilt" because their lives have been spared.

Whatever the reasons for the guilt, most guilt feelings are based on irrational assumptions. Usually, in reality, there was nothing more anyone could humanly have done. There are times, nonetheless, when guilt is real and culpable. Thus, the young man who left his seriously ailing mother alone on the night she died and spent the night partying with friends may justifiably feel a sense of guilt. This guilt, like others, needs to be confronted and resolved.

In processing a loss the bereaved run the gamut of emotions as they realize the impact of the loss and recognize the changes they will need to make and face in their lives. The meaning and realization of the loss unfolds with each encounter and experience without the deceased. There are those who say that, unless one has experienced such a loss, the impact is difficult to imagine.

Phase Three – Resolution

The final phase of grief begins when the bereaved begins the process of reorganizing his or her life to adjust to life without the deceased. Grieving is timeless and there are no norms to follow. Some people report waking up one morning and making the conscious decision to pull their lives together. Others have reported that one day they realized suddenly that the pain was not as intense and that they had started healing. Others have needed to be encouraged to move into the final stages of grieving. And, unfortunately, there are some who, years after the death, still have difficulty resolving the loss.

When a bereaved wife can reflect on her deceased husband with fond feelings mingled with sadness, rather than sharp pain and intense longing, and when she can accept both her negative and positive feelings for him, then she has begun to resolve and adjust to the loss. Individuals in this phase recognize that life must continue without the deceased. Therefore, they begin socializing and resume interest in everyday activities. They may identify new goals or continue working towards future goals. Life is experienced again as ordered, meaningful, and with a sense of purpose.

Many bereaved persons report gradually regaining their hope and strength during the final phase of grieving. Because they feel they are resolving their loss, they tend to experience a feeling of pride, not unlike a recovering addict, for having made it through the worst. It is a myth to think that, once the bereaved have reached this stage, they no longer experience waves of sadness. Anniversaries, holidays, a song may still reawaken the feelings of loss. However, the memories begin to be reflected on as bitter-sweet ones.

Grieving in order to resolve a loss is not an arbitrary process. As Colin Murray Parkes poignantly stated: "The pain of grief is as much a part of life as the joy of love; it is the price we pay for love, it is the cost of commitment" (Murray Parkes 1974, p. 5).

Thus, if we did not love, we would not grieve. Grieving a loss is never ever completed, but with time, we can not only live with the sense of loss but also grow as a result of it.

CHAPTER 2

The Social and Psychological Effects of Loss

In chapter one, the pain of bereavement was examined from an intrapsychic and psychological perspective. However, the effects of loss are also experienced interpersonally as most losses occur within the context of a family unit where some type of homeostatic balance exists. A significant loss will disrupt that balance and can cause impaired relationships that extend not just within but outside of the family unit. When working with bereaved individuals, therefore, it is important to have some knowledge of the roles played by various persons with whom they interact as well as the relationships that are hindering or facilitating grieving.

A common source of interpersonal difficulties is when there is displacement of feelings, that is, the bereaved find it difficult to vent feelings directly at whom they feel is responsible and instead vent at a substitute source. Additionally unresolved grief may be "carried over" from one generation to the next and affect relationships. When this occurs, the conflicts in the present family relationships actually have their origin in the past.

A student in an undergraduate psychology course I once taught wrote a story on the effects of separation, though I had not instructed her to do so. The story is . . .

Life Is Not a Bed of Roses

A Short Story
By Nikola Nolan

The phrase "life is not a bed of roses" is one big understatement that I have come to understand. People who have minor difficulties use this phrase lightly but I think I should buy the copyright so it would only be used in my situation, as the better part of my youth has been sheer hell.

It all began when my comfortable little world crumbled because the two people I admired and respected most were no longer the loving couple I once knew. They snapped and snapped at each other until the little bit which was holding them together snapped in two. And that was the end, or should I say the beginning of my life of sheer hell.

The separation of my parents hit me like a ton of bricks! I tried to throw off the awful pain it inflicted upon me by wishing I was as young and naive as my little five year old sister. She thought Daddy was not coming home because he had "passed on", which was the only answer my Mom could find to give Shauna.

I must admit, the separation affected my Mom severely too. It reached the point where her parenting practices became non-existent. Our once beautiful relationship now turned into that of a forceful slave master and an ill-treated slave. She became totally insensitive to my needs, and I just did not know how to deal with this new monster of a mother.

Anyway, at that time, I could not care less about Mommy's pain. All I could think about was me and the fact that a fifteen year old did not deserve to have this big messy load shoved down her throat. Just when the world was proving to be a wonderful place and Dwight from next door had just started to show a little interest in me. Anyway, might as well he had kept his over-sized nose in the air, as he usually does when he passes me by, because this separation had changed me. It reached the point where one day I knocked a smile off Dwight's face and sent him flying in a pool of water with his nose right back in the air.

I just could not understand why he was so bright and chirpy with this beaming smile as if life was a bowl of strawberry ice cream. As far as I was concerned, life was the pits, so the comprehension of his mood was totally beyond me.

It is all well and good for you to sit there and say "Poor Dwight, he did not deserve that." But what about me? After all it was I who had to rush home to collect my sister from school and cook dinner because Mom was holding down two jobs in order to keep us alive. Not to mention the fact that the cleaning and washing automatically became my duties because my now disgusting Mom says she now foots the bills so I had better play my part. This was very hard for me, especially when I thought about the fact that I should be out there living it up with my friends. Instead I was struggling with all this household work like an old maid.

I must admit that by now I did not have many friends since the likes of me just could not stand to hear them bragging about their perfect little mummies and daddies. Eventually, I detached myself from my peers and trod slowly in my now one-man gang. Even until this day I am still anti-social and full of anger and pain. But it no longer affects Dwight from next door. It now affects Paul. Dear sweet Paul who loves me so much and wishes to marry me. But I just cannot relate to him properly, not to mention marrying him. I will not give this divorce thing a chance to hit me directly. Oh no! I have had my fair share.

There is another thing. Paul just chats on and on about his happy childhood. He is ignorant of mine because of my choice to keep it to myself. Still, I hate him for it. Although I should not, I cannot help it. That is just me, bitter, bitter as gall.

Looking back now I can say there was a little good that came out of the separation. When Dad began visiting, he would shower me with love and attention and not to mention money. In the long run, however, that was no good because the attention did not ease the pain or remove the keloids left by the terrible wounds of having my heart torn apart. Even the money was no fun after a while. Can you believe that? Well you see there were no friends to blow it with. Wow! What can I say? Life is certainly no bed of roses. Trust me.

The effects of divorce on interpersonal relationships, described in the story, can be, and have been, mirrored in individuals who have recently migrated and left behind family, friends and security. It is also seen in the bereaved whose loved ones have died.

Regardless of the circumstances of a major loss, persons should be helped to identify and understand the gamut of their feelings. This will help them to be better prepared to deal with the many practical and social changes that will occur in everyday life; changes that will make life feel topsy-turvy initially. These changes include taking on more responsibility and roles within the home, learning domestic skills, getting a second job, assuming responsibility for paying utility bills, balancing a checkbook, acquiring a driver's license, adjusting to loss of financial assets or income, redefining social interests or activities.

Not only does a loss upset the equilibrium of those facing it, but it can also disrupt interpersonal bonds. Both the mother and teenaged daughter in the story appear to feel that no one will be able to understand their pain. Hence, there is a forced isolation of self and an often subconscious egocentrism or insensitivity to the feelings of others. Such reactions can create bewilderment, confusion, and anger in friends, relatives, and coworkers.

Grieving a loss therefore has many implications. While there are intrapsychic feelings to attend to, there are also practical, social, and interpersonal changes with which to reckon.

CHAPTER 3

Bereavement Outcomes

What Are my Options?

The bereaved will make one of three choices during the course of his or her grief:

1. To carry out the often unconscious desire to die
2. To remain in mourning, because it requires too much energy to make the necessary life adjustments
3. To relinquish the past and move forward

The Choice to Die
The first choice is seldom discussed because of the taboo placed on causing one's own death. However, the high mortality rate among elderly bereaved spouses suggests that the bereaved may indeed be choosing to die. North American statistics indicate that the highest rate of suicide in the entire US population is among white men over the age of 85 years (Papalia and Olds 1992).

Older people who take their own lives seem to plan carefully, as one out of every two reported suicide attempts in old age is successful. Despair over a series of irreversible losses, not only of a spouse, but of work, friends, children and health seems to culminate in the severe feeling of hopelessness leading to suicide. Interestingly, in 1993 in the USA, the media brought attention to a medical practitioner in Michigan who became known as the "suicide doctor" or Dr "Death" because he was granting persons with an incurable illness their wish by helping them to die.

The accuracy of the incidence of suicide in the elderly is unclear because sometimes the deaths are ruled as accidental, from drug overdose, traffic accidents, or forgetting to take medication. One study conducted in a semirural community in Wales (Rees and Lutkins 1967) found that within the first year following loss the mortality rate among surviving spouses was 12.2 percent. This number was halved by the second year and further reduced by the third year. In light of these statistics, medical practitioners should be careful of prescribing tranquilizers and other medication to the recently bereaved, especially the elderly.

The Choice to Remain in Mourning
Grief that does not get resolved is termed abnormal, pathological or complicated. There are three main forms of complicated reactions in which the bereaved continue to mourn. These are classified as chronic, delayed and masked grief. In a chronic grief situation the bereaved's grief is prolonged and excessive in duration. Although mourning a loss is considered timeless, when individuals find themselves grieving physically and emotionally for several years and the pain is still acute, the grief process has become complicated. The bereaved can know when their reaction is chronic because they feel they are not getting on with their lives. Of

the three forms of pathological reactions, those who are experiencing chronic grief are most likely to seek professional help.

The term "delayed reaction" would suggest that no grief was initially displayed by the bereaved at the time of the loss. In reality, however, it is often the case that the bereaved person does show some emotions briefly, but feels that the response was inappropriate or "not sufficient" for the loss. When this occurs the bereaved person may grieve excessively over a subsequent loss or over the primary loss at a future date.

Delayed reactions can be triggered vicariously through, for example, watching someone crying on the television. More commonly, however, a delayed reaction is triggered when someone experiences multiple losses, which incidentally are not limited to death. A recent loss can therefore reawaken unresolved feelings from a previous loss and cause an exaggerated reaction. Persons whose grief reactions are delayed may seek help to cope with their losses because of their perception that their grief is inappropriate for the present loss.

It is seldom that the bereaved whose grief is masked will voluntarily seek psychological counselling. This is unfortunate, because these persons are the most likely to be helped by professional counselling. In masked grief there are no overt signs of grieving but the bereaved will experience symptoms and behaviours that interfere with their effective functioning. These individuals develop non-affective symptoms such as physical aches and pains, but fail to recognize the relationship between their symptoms and the loss.

Masked reactions are formed at the unconscious level. Persons who did not allow themselves to grieve can develop, for example, ulcers, headaches and psychosomatic disorders. At times the symptoms can be similar to those that the deceased relative had. Because we have been socialized to accept physical pain as more "real" than psychological pain, physical pain can be used to mask grief. Conduct disorders such as fire setting in children and self-destructive acts such as drug addiction can be other forms of masked reactions that are not easily recognized as grief-related behaviours.

The Choice to Move Forward
The bereaved person who is motivated to move forward through the grieving experience has accepted the meaning of the loss, both intellectually and emotionally, and has validated and ventilated his or her feelings. With the help of friends, family, pastor or counsellor the bereaved may be encouraged to reflect, for example, on the circumstances surrounding the loss and the good and bad memories shared with the deceased. This helps them to actualize the loss and accommodate it in their lives. There are persons, nonetheless, who prefer to say their goodbyes and reflect on the memories by themselves. Whichever route the bereaved person takes, one of the necessary tasks in moving forward is saying goodbye to the deceased.

The bereaved also need to have their feelings validated by others and to be given the opportunity to vent them, if they so desire. Some may be troubled about expressing their feelings because they feel there is nonacceptance by others when they express negative emotions. Some may feel that they are burdening their families and friends when they express fear and anxiety. Others may feel that expressing feelings of helplessness or insecurity is admitting to failure, signs of weakness and immaturity.

Although family, friends, acquaintances and counsellors would not intentionally discourage the expression of grief, unfortunately this has not always been communicated to the bereaved. Getting their feelings validated and feeling comfortable in expressing their grief are important tasks for the bereaved who are working through their grief.

A loss will bring about changes in the life of surviving family members, and at times these changes may be difficult to manage. Financial woes, feelings of loneliness and other problems arise which demand that the bereaved utilize effective problem solving techniques. This may not be easy initially, as the judgement and decision making skills of the bereaved are likely to be affected by their grieving.

As a general rule, the bereaved are advised not to make any major life changes immediately following a loss. For example, they should not relocate, change careers or jobs, or remarry too soon after the death event. The bereaved need stability, emotional support and to be around the familiar at this time. Any major changes therefore may be counterproductive to them moving forward with their grief. Although the advice of friends and supporters is welcome, it is important that the bereaved perceive themselves as making their own decisions. This will encourage them to feel "I will survive, I am going to make it."

According to William Worden (1982), a noted grief counsellor, the final task the bereaved has to accomplish in the grieving process is that of forming new relationships.

Worden believes the bereaved need to withdraw the emotional energy they had invested in their relationship with the deceased and reinvest this energy in another relationship. This task is often misconstrued because it is misinterpreted to mean that the bereaved must forget about the deceased. This is not being suggested, however, as it is not possible to forget about our loved ones.

When survivors invest in a new relationship they are taking on new commitments and this encourages them to carry on living and loving. The young lady in the story told in the previous chapter needed to have heeded that advice. Unfortunately, there are many popular love songs that propagate the myth that, when a loved one dies, the person left behind will not be able to find love again.

CHAPTER 4

Theoretical Explanations of Grief

Why Is Grief so Painful at Times?

In this chapter the diverse ways in which man responds to and copes with bereavement are examined from sociocultural, medical, and religious perspectives.

The Sociocultural Perspective

My experience as a Jamaican living in Aberdeen, Scotland definitely shaped my thoughts on the importance of culture in influencing the outcome of the bereavement experience. I can recall when the father of one of my colleagues died. I approached my colleague and offered my condolences verbally and with a card. He informed me in a polite but curt manner that my expressions were not necessary and that he would prefer if everyone quickly returned to "life as usual". It was later explained to me by other Aberdonians that it was typical for them not to display or have others display open expressions of sorrow. That experience helped to shape my PhD dissertation on bereavement. I examined loss from a cultural perspective and developed an ethnofocal theory and model to try and explain the different grief experiences.

In my thesis I attempted to show that culture affects the grief process in two primary ways. First, each person has a personal code of grief reaction; that is, a personal belief system which dictates how to react to a loss. This belief system or code is dependent on the family's beliefs and/or the social rules and norms of the immediate social network within which the individual was brought up. This personal code is what or who we are at any given time and is closely associated with an individual's sense of self.

Secondly, each person is subjected to a societal code, which reflects the informal rules of the society at large on how to behave during bereavement. These rules are the cultural values, attitudes and traditions that distinguish one society from another. The societal code can be totally adopted, thus becoming synonymous to the personal code, or it can be partially adopted or not adopted at all.

The relationship between these two codes (personal and societal) determines one's response to the death of a loved one. When the personal code of a bereaved person is similar to that of the societal code, he or she will feel free to choose how to respond to the loss. In this situation the bereaved person would not be unduly anxious about whether his or her behaviours conform to societal norms.

On the other hand, when both codes are at variance, dissonance occurs, and this can compound the stress of the experience for the bereaved. This latter scenario arises, for example, when individuals migrate to another country. The transplanted individuals may feel that their traditional style of expressing grief is not accepted by the members of their social circle in the "adopted" country. Consequently, they may experience dissonance between their personal code of grief reaction and the societal code, and thus may feel pressured to modify their grief response.

Case studies and observations were used to test the premise of my theory. The results indicated that an ethnofocal theory on grief can provide guidelines as to what behaviours can be expected of bereaved individuals of different sociocultural backgrounds (Pottinger 1990).

Generally, the research indicated that those who are brought up to openly express their grief feelings are likely to do so satisfactorily during bereavement. However, those who feel this behaviour is not socially appropriate and yet openly grieve run the risk of being additionally distressed about the loss. Also, individuals who are brought up in a society that sanctions the non-expression of grief appear to cope effectively if they continue to control or suppress their grief feelings during bereavement.

Other researchers have examined how the attitudes and beliefs of the family are critical in influencing how one responds to a loss. For example, Pine (1989) has shown how family members and friends can either encourage or discourage the expression of grief by their verbal and nonverbal communication.

Health professionals may also unintentionally influence the grief response of their bereaved patients or clients. A doctor who is feeling uncomfortable about his or her own mortality or who feels helpless in assisting a patient may use psychological tactics to distance him- or herself from the patient. When doctors are quick to prescribe sedatives or are too busy to talk with their patients, bereaved patients may feel that their doctors are discouraging them from expressing their grief. Kane and colleagues (1985), in a study conducted in the USA, found that increased communication between bereaved family members and their doctors resulted in a significant decline in reports of anxiety and distress by the recently bereaved.

The Medical Perspective
Traditionally, when the recently bereaved have sought help for coping with loss they have been diagnosed as either depressed or "under stress" and treated accordingly.

The Depression Model
Health workers in the 1960s described the grief response to a loved one's death as a physical illness. Grief was likened to an illness because it (1) involves impairment of capacity to function; (2) has a predictable course and set of symptoms; and (3) has a known aetiology (Engel 1961). In addition, many of the symptoms that are present in the recently bereaved closely resemble the cluster of symptoms associated with a diagnosis of depression. In both presentations there is sleep disturbance, feelings of hopelessness and anxiety, spells of crying, inertia, reduction of activities or agitated activity. Because of the relatedness between grief reaction and reactive depression, depression has been widely used as a model for understanding grief.

John Bowlby, a major contributor to research on attachment attempted to explain the "depressed" reaction to loss in his thesis on attachment and loss (Bowlby 1969). He suggested that attachment is a primordial response in humans. We constantly strive to belong to someone, a group or belief system which will provide us with security and a base for exploring novel situations. Thus, when we are prevented from maintaining a sense of security with a significant attachment figure this is antithetic to man's nature. According to Bowlby the result is mental anguish, despair and depression.

When a mother is temporarily removed from the presence of her baby, the baby responds with anxiety and cries of apparent distress. Babies have not had the opportunity to learn this response, yet they all act similarly. Bowlby feels, therefore, that grieving is both a biological and sociological response. He has helped us to understand why the loss of a mother, who is usually the first source of bonding for the infant, is traumatic to the bereaved of any age.

When a loved one dies, a vacuum is created because of the various roles that the deceased had filled. Thus, the husband who loses his wife may have lost a friend, partner in business, lover, listener, domestic help-mate, teacher and decision maker. It is the multiplicity of these roles that are now lost that exaggerate the feelings of hopelessness, anxiety and other depressive symptoms experienced during grief.

When the bereaved loses motivation and drive to relate to others and withdraws from social activities, the pain of loss is prolonged. Becoming socially withdrawn robs the bereaved of the emotional support that he or she needs at this time to counteract feelings of hopelessness and isolation. In addition, the reduction of activities provides the bereaved person with much time to reminisce on the loss and remain in mourning.

At the time of a loss there is a renewed awareness that man has no power over controlling death. Subsequently, the bereaved may lose their sense of direction and feel overwhelmed by their sense of powerlessness. Psychologists describe this response as a state of "learned helplessness" (Seligman 1972). Usually this state is temporary. However, when it is prolonged the feelings of hopelessness, vulnerability and cognitive disorganization that are generated can cause severe depression and anxiety.

The stress model

Can one die of a broken heart? A husband and wife team of psychologists, M. Stroebe and W. Stroebe (1987), have assembled a comprehensive review of what is known about the impact of bereavement on surviving marital partners. They have suggested that stress and depression are part of the same phenomenon. When stress is added to grief, depression is likely to develop. The Stroebes believe that the multiple losses, both tangible and intangible, that are incurred when a loved one dies result in major changes in the life of the bereaved. When there is loss or change, there is the potential for stress.

Kastenbaum (1985) coined the term "bereavement overload" to explain the stress reaction he observed in the bereaved. He found that individuals who had social and economic problems tended to perceive the death of a loved one as another burden. The cumulative experience led to feelings of hopelessness and helplessness. A study I conducted at a hospice center in Jamaica support these findings (Pottinger and Alexander 1990). Those relatives who were from a lower socioeconomic bracket were more likely than those from a higher socioeconomic bracket to report feelings of numbness, shock and distress after the death of a loved one.

Over the past 40 years researchers have been documenting the impact that the death of a close relative can have on survivors. Some studies have suggested that the death of a significant other increases the risk of death from coronary disease in the next of kin (Jenkins 1971). There are also reports by Kaprio et al. (1987) supporting an increase in the mortality rate among the recently bereaved for the first month of bereavement. Do these findings suggest therefore that one can die of a broken heart?

Selye (1976) in his book, *The Stress of Life*, describes the physiological effect that excessive stress has on the body. The body's response is threefold: there is (1) enlargement of the adrenal cortex; (2) shrinkage of the thymus, spleen, lymph nodes and other lymphatic structures; and (3) bleeding and ulcers in the lining of the stomach. Stress does not have a direct impact on the functioning of the heart muscle. However, the glands and structures that are affected are related to the functioning of the body's immune defenses and cardiovascular system.

The physiological impact of stress on the body should not be automatically construed as debilitating. It is only when the stress is prolonged and exceeds the body's ability to adapt that it becomes harmful. Also, if the body was already in a weakened state then the physiological changes could break down the already weakened system.

Labelling bereavement as distressing is related more to one's perception of the events as stressful rather than the actual death event itself. Research experts on stress (Folkman et al. 1986) have concluded that stress is a particular relationship between a person and his or her environment, which can be perceived by the person as taxing or exceeding his or her resources.

From my research and experience with the bereaved I have found that those who do not appraise the stress of bereavement as harmful are those who (1) have a stable, non-neurotic personality; (2) feel that they are equipped with the necessary coping skills; (3) feel that they have access to emotional and social support from family and friends.

The Religious–Philosophical Perspective

There is some evidence indicating that having strong religious faith enhances one's ability to cope with a major loss such as bereavement (Murray Parkes 1986). It is suggested that being spiritual or religious enables one to take advantage of religious rituals and support during this time. Thielman and Melges (1986) have also proposed that religion helps to redefine the loss for the bereaved and gives them a "language" from which to draw comfort for their pain.

Religion is believed to help the bereaved in three main ways. One of its purposes is psychological as it provides a framework for the bereaved to express their grief. Mourning is sanctioned in the Bible. In Matthew 5: 4 (according to the King James version), Jesus said *"Blessed are they that mourn for they shall be comforted."* Ecclesiastes 7: 4 reads, *"For by mourning is a man's soul made better."* Various personalities are portrayed in the Bible crying, including Jesus (Luke 19: 41). The impression is given, therefore, that grieving is necessary and accepted and is a temporary state from which one progresses with the grace of God.

A second function provided by religion is a sociological one. When a loved one dies there is usually a religious ritual or ceremony, such as a funeral, where family, friends and the community can gather and offer consolation to the bereaved and say prayers for the deceased.

These rituals vary according to one's culture but the intent is usually supportive. For Irish families, death is considered a big event and the family will go to great lengths to give the dead a good "send off". The tradition is to have an all night vigil on the night before the burial in the presence of the corpse which is not to be left alone until burial. This famous Irish vigil is known as the wake. Traditionally, wakes are merry events, where family members of the deceased gather and tell stories and jokes, are likely to get drunk, and there is generally a party-like atmosphere. The best that one can say about a successful wake is that the deceased would have enjoyed it.

Jews also have a set of rituals related to burying their dead. One such is the tradition of a meal prepared by neighbours and eaten ceremoniously in the home of the bereaved. This ritual is referred to as the "first meal of restoration" and is the first full meal following a Jewish burial (Yodder 1986). It signifies the restoring of strength and faith to the surviving family members.

In Jamaica, a blending of African and Christian traditions can be observed in traditional funeral rituals. When someone dies a "set 'n up" or wake is held every night until the day of the funeral. This wake is referred to as "nine night" (Pigou 1987). Inside the house of the deceased a light is kept burning for nine nights because it is believed that the spirit of the dead person returns to its home on the ninth night after the death. Jamaicans will then arrange a service on the ninth night. This service is open to the community and can include hymn singing, a speech by a leader, foot stomping, the serving of refreshments, and playing of dominoes and cards.

In all these communal acts, and many others, the bereaved get an opportunity to vent their feelings and to receive comfort and support from a wide network of people. These traditional rituals, however, are fast fading as there is a growing cynicism about religion and religious rituals. In fact elaborate funerals are gradually being replaced by quick, "sophisticated" ceremonies. Some researchers believe that these changes are resulting in an increasing number of bereaved persons finding it difficult to cope with their loss. They argue that this is because the bereaved no longer have access to the communal spirit and support and the public sanctioning of grief provided by the rituals (Gorer 1965).

The third function provided by religion is that it offers a theological or philosophical explanation of the death. For example, Christian theologians believe that man is made up of three parts, the body, the spirit and the soul (First Thessalonians 5: 23). When a man dies his body is the only part that dies and goes back to dust. The spirit, which is the God-filled part of man, and the soul, which animates the body while alive, do not die.

Christians argue that it makes a difference whether or not a person dies as a believer in God. Believers are taught that, as Christ ascended into heaven, so will they go in the presence of the Lord when they die. Death is therefore not seen as the end, but a new beginning (1 Corinthians 15).

Bereaved Christians can draw comfort and a feeling of peace at the death of a loved one. They believe that their loved one is "better off" and happy, as they are now free from sin and at rest from their labours and struggles (Romans 6: 7).

They also believe that those who "die knowing the Lord" will not know torment (Luke 16: 24) because they have escaped the fate of sinners.

Although Christianity is the only religion cited in this section of the book, readers are referred to writings on other religions which also provide for believers a framework for accepting the loss, and from which they can draw comfort and strength (see Walsh and McGoldrich 1991).

CHAPTER 5

Bereavement in Childhood

Is it Different for Children?

Many parents report feeling uncertain about how and when to help their bereaved children. The need to provide answers for these children and knowledge to their caregivers is becoming increasingly evident as the levels of crime and violence in societies continue to rise. In the USA, in the inner cities and among ethnic minorities 1 in 21 African Americans between the ages of 14 and 34 years has a chance of becoming a homicide victim. This was documented in a survey of high schools done in an inner city where forty percent of the children had a family member or friend who had died by homicide (Greene 1993). A similar situation exists in Jamaica and Scotland where crime statistics are high and death by violence ranks among the top three leading causes of death.

In spite of the statistics, these societies are still relatively "closed" on the subject of children and bereavement. Many adults try to protect their children from being exposed to death by, for example, preventing them from participating in the funeral ceremony or not allowing the children to see them grieve. This "protection" has also been witnessed in other forms of loss, such as migration. It is a common experience for Jamaican parents not to prepare their children for the imminent separation when they are migrating to another country. Parents will describe that they want to protect their children from the sadness and anxiety of the departure.

According to Teresa Rando, a well known expert in the field, not assisting the bereaved child to actively confront a loss is to predispose the child to pathology and life-long problems (Rando 1984). Thus, if a funeral ceremony can help to promote realization and confirmation of a loss it will be therapeutic for the child to participate in it.

Normally, adults use much emotional strength during grief because it is not easy for them to begin life anew without the loved one who has died. Imagine then the struggle in the young child, who does not have the necessary cognitive skills and behavioural coping strategies to overcome the wish to remain closely connected to the deceased.

Children's understanding and response to death differ depending on a number of factors. These include their age, developmental stage, cognitive level of functioning, emotional health and social circumstances. By age two, a child's play can demonstrate an awareness of loss. However, child specialists believe that preschoolers have not as yet developed the cognitive skills to understand death. They view death as temporary and reversible, but this is not to say that they will not respond to the loss they are feeling.

From about five years of age, a child begins to realize the finality of death. Initially they think of death as something that happens to others but gradually they begin to realize that one day it will also happen to them. Despite this growing understanding, however, a child is still unable to fully understand and cope with the reality of death, as adults do, until they are approaching their tenth birthday. In fact some researchers believe that children between the ages of five to seven years are particularly at risk for a poor adjustment to loss. During these years the child can cognitively understand, for example, the irreversibility and finality of death but they are still not emotionally able to cope with the meaning of the loss (Worden 1982).

The child who is not emotionally prepared to cope with a loss will not be able to experience the cathartic release adults get when they cry or express their feelings. Some researchers who have thoroughly studied the reactions of children to parental loss report behavioural changes rather than affective symptoms as being typical. For example, Worden (1982) and Raphael (1984) found that bereaved children will temporarily have disturbed sleep such as nightmares, and will display aggressive, withdrawn or clinging behaviours. They also noted a sharp decline in academic interest and performance and a corresponding increase in interest in non-school related activities. A depressive syndrome comprising sadness, irritability, poor school performance and nightmares has been reported in both sexes but more prevalently in older girls (Bentovin 1986).

Adolescents are another age group of persons who are particularly prone to developing complicated grief reactions. It is possible that the transitional nature of the adolescents' development and their perception of immortality heightens their vulnerability and risk. Many of the bereaved adolescents with whom I have worked have either been explicitly angry at themselves or the world or have tried to mask their anger. Anger is common because death is such a shock to their system that it adds to the turmoil and confusion they are already experiencing from the regular stresses of growing up.

When adolescents turn the anger inward on themselves, this can result in self-destructive behaviours, such as addiction, promiscuity and also depression. For many adolescents bereavement goes awry because their anger has not been dealt with and expressed. Another maladaptive coping strategy that is common to adolescents is when they idealize the lost relationship. Adolescents can rewrite history in their minds and become preoccupied with ideal fantasies about the deceased and the relationship they had with them. This fantasizing is maladaptive, as it can prevent them from moving on and investing in new relationships.

Of all the losses a child can experience, parental loss has been the most extensively studied. In a study of bereaved children under five years, Colin Murray Parkes described how these children tended to manifest excessive clinging behaviours, jealousy and temper tantrums when faced with the loss of a caregiver (Murray Parkes 1965). Because there is no real understanding of the meaning of loss for them, however, the permanence of their reactions is dependent on the responses of their surviving parents and guardians. The failure of adults to cope with the loss themselves and to meet the needs of their children will affect the child's ability to cope with the present loss and also his or her ability to form deep attachments in the future (Bentovin 1986).

There is a subtle norm that acknowledges a child's loss of

his or her parent but prevents the child from mourning the loss of a sibling. Children are often not given the opportunity to vent their feelings of guilt, fear, loneliness and anger when a sibling dies. In many cases even when brothers and sisters share a close relationship they are not always loving with each other. Birth order, differences in academic performance and differences in physical appearance can cause rivalry among siblings. When a sibling dies, therefore, there may be conflicting or ambivalent feelings, which can complicate the grief process. Sibling death has also been known to result in the survivor experiencing "survivor guilt", the feeling that the "nicer child" has died (Sanders 1989).

In a study done in the late 1960s, it was shown that a half of the sample of children who had experienced the death of a sibling by leukemia had poor adjustment both to the illness and after the loss. The surviving siblings, who were previously well emotionally, displayed symptoms of acute onset of enuresis (bed wetting), headaches, poor school performance, school phobia, depression and anxiety (Binger et al. 1969).

It is important to note that, in earlier studies particularly, the reports on children's grief were made mainly by their parents who themselves were grieving. The reports therefore could be biased and reflect the parents' grief. Nonetheless, children will model their parents and exhibit similar responses. Thus, parents and guardians need to be careful that they are allowing their children to freely express their grief and that they are not doing anything to either prolong or interfere with their child's grief process.

The importance of helping a child to accept and grieve a loss cannot be overstated. Adults can discuss the loss with the child, as this helps the child to put words to his or her feelings. The adult can also use that opportunity to convey to the child his or her acceptance of the death and faith in the future.

Adult family members who feel uncomfortable speaking about loss to their child may use books or films on bereavement to assist them. Reading a book or having a book read may lead a child to ask relevant questions about the loss and to confront his or her thoughts, fears and feelings. Books can offer insights into expected feelings and reassure the child about his or her reactions. They can provide information about difficult periods such as holidays and anniversaries, and suggest coping strategies that are age appropriate. However, reading a book should not be used as a replacement for verbal discussion but as a facilitator.

Even with assistance there will still be some family members who will not feel able or prepared at that time to help a child grieve his or her loss. These individuals should not be made to feel inadequate or guilty. Instead their feelings should be accepted and the bereaved child could be referred to a professional counsellor.

CHAPTER 6

Suicide

Why Didn't she Say Goodbye?

The US and Jamaican media have brought attention to the steady increase in suicide rate in these two countries, especially by adolescents. In fact the American Psychological Association dedicated the February 1993 issue of the *American Psychologist* journal to research on adolescence and suicide. Many people find life so precious that they cannot understand why anyone would voluntarily end it. Yet the 1988 official US data (National Center for Health Statistics) indicated that, on average, one suicide occurs every 17.3 minutes.

US epidemiological statistics reveal that males are three to four times more likely to commit suicide than females, although females do attempt suicide more often. Those who are over 45 years have the highest rate, especially if they are older than 75 years. In absolute numbers, however, most suicide victims are found within the ages of 15 to 34 years. The divorced and widowed have been found to be statistically at risk, as well as those who are unemployed or employed as medical doctors. Other population groups that have a comparatively high incidence of suicide are whites and persons of Asian descent, as well as immigrants in their adopted countries.

In addition to these demographic data, there are other factors that heighten the risk of individuals committing suicide. Persons who have had psychiatric treatment, who are schizophrenic or prone to depression, who are addicted to drugs, whether illegal drugs or prescribed ones or those who have a major or chronic illness are at risk for suicide.

The best single predictor of suicide is a previous suicide attempt. Studies show that up to forty percent of those who try to commit suicide will make more than one attempt, and that ten percent to fifteen percent of repeaters will be successful (Garland and Zigler 1993). About half of those who have attempted suicide will talk about it.

A small percentage of suicide victims communicate verbally their intention to commit suicide. Nevertheless, in eight out of ten cases some warning signs are given. Personality changes, such as apathy or unusual anger, signs of depression, such as neglect of appearance, difficulty concentrating at work or school, feelings of helplessness or hopelessness, anxiety and sudden withdrawal from family and friends, can all be warning signals. Additionally, talking about death, suicide or life hereafter and giving away prized possessions can be considered warnings. Statisticians have found, for reasons not fully understood, that most suicides occur during the spring season, or the months March, April and May, as well as during significant holidays or family anniversaries.

There are certain personality traits that cause a person to be vulnerable to taking his or her life. Low self-esteem, resulting in frequent bouts of depression, usually underlies the "suicider's" personality. These persons also tend to be dependent and have poor problem solving skills. A review of the literature shows the typical suicide victim as being immature, manipulative, feeling psychologically alone and having a low self-esteem with inadequate or rigid defenses. The use of a firearm is the most common method of committing suicide for both genders. This is followed by hanging for males and ingestion of drugs for females.

Researchers, such as Kastenbaum and Aisenberg (1976), who have studied the subject of suicide, suggest that the suicide victim's low self-esteem is related to chronic feelings of insecurity arising from either real or perceived abandonment or rejection during childhood. In later adult life, these persons seem to unconsciously seek out experiences resulting in failure and rejection, thus reinforcing their low self-esteem. They also tend to over-respond to crises when they arise.

Most of the information that has been gathered about suicide victims has been obtained, for obvious reasons, either from those who unsuccessfully attempted suicide or from those who have not actually attempted suicide, but have appealed for help because they were having suicidal thoughts. In addition, a "psychological autopsy" can be performed on a suicide victim whereby, after the act has been committed, attempts are made to reconstruct the life of the victim through the recollections of family members and friends. This method has been used frequently with adolescents, resulting in the identification of drug and alcohol abuse, prior suicide attempt, depression, family history of suicidal behaviours and availability of a firearm as being the most common risk factors among this age group (Garland and Zigler 1993).

Suicide carries a social stigma and is frightening to the public. People are fearful of hearing about a healthy, robust person losing control of his or her life to the extent that he or she engages in the ultimate act of self destruction. Some suicide acts can be deliberately committed and others are passive, whereby the person's inaction results in a failure to preserve his or her life.

Some explanations that have been offered for suicide are that the victims:

1. Were in such discomfort and pain that their only goal was to escape the pain
2. Believed that the future was going to be no better than the present, or it would be worse
3. Were impulsive and had not thought about the future
4. Believed they were dying
5. Were mentally ill and did not know what they were doing
6. Felt that what could be gained symbolically through death was more important than what life had to offer

It is my understanding that a person's perspective of time becomes distorted when he or she is attempting suicide. The individual loses his or her sense of continuity of time and the ability to think of alternative solutions. One person who had attempted suicide described to me that during those moments when she attempted to take her life, she felt as if the walls of the room were closing in on her and there was no alternative solution but to cease to feel. At that moment she could not and did not think of her children or the future because she had lost her sense of time. There was no past or future for her, just the present moment.

Adolescent Suicide

A review of books, journals and the media over the past two decades indicates that adolescent suicide is steadily increasing. One researcher in the US has claimed that between 1960 and 1988 the suicide rate among adolescents rose by 200 percent, compared to a general population increase of 17 percent (Garland and Zigler 1993). In Canada, the US and the UK suicide is ranked within the top three causes of death within this age group. It is possible that the increased attention to suicide is resulting in more medical examiners labelling sudden deaths as suicide rather than an accident, hence the increase in numbers. However, on the other hand, it is also the case that statistics on suicide are usually under-represented because of the social stigma that is associated with this type of loss.

A few years ago a seventeen-year-old mother of a baby girl refused counselling despite her mother's pleas and concerns about their turbulent mother-daughter relationship. The seventeen-year-old had a history of promiscuity and running away from home. One year after the initial counselling interview with the mother, the daughter was found dead of a drug overdose. A nine-year-old boy, whose father had died recently, tearfully tells his mother one night, some months after the death, that he is depressed and is thinking of killing himself. A nineteen-year-old youth rushes home angrily after being involved in a car accident, grabs his gun and shoots himself in the head.

These three incidents occurred in Jamaica, but are no different from the thousands of stories told in the US or UK

What is it that makes life so intolerable for people who are so young? Some child specialists believe that children are being put under too much stress to achieve academic excellence, be popular among their peers, be a leader and to conform, all at once. Added to that, parental acceptance and love are given contingently on the child's social and academic success. Additionally, proessionals who study child development believe that today's youths are under too much pressure to acquire adult responsibilities at an early age (Elkind 1984). In single parent homes and homes where parents are unable to model effective parenting skills, children are being given responsibilities of parenting and taking care of younger siblings as well as running a home. Hence, contemporary society with its educational and social demands is seen as forcing children to grow up too quickly.

Technological and other advances which are aimed at making societies more civilized and sophisticated are also indirectly blamed for the increase in adolescent suicide. Contemporary families are more mobile, thus disrupting community bonding and the "protective" support of the extended family system. Also, Western societies are felt to be undermining the development of an adequate control system in children through its often wrongly interpreted teachings of "freedom of expression" and its modelling of life "in the fast lane" (Kastenbaum and Aisenberg 1976).

The increase in availability of firearms to teens and easy access to drugs have also been identified as contributing factors to the high adolescent suicide rate. In fact Garland and Zigler (1993) found that approximately one third of adolescent "suiciders" were intoxicated at the time of their death.

Other common methods of committing suicide is by wrist-cutting, jumping and reckless driving. The method of choice seems to be dependent on accessibility to, and familiarity with, the tool, the individual's state of mind and the meaning and cultural significance of the method. Common precipitants include trouble at home, arguments, disappointment and humiliation.

Intervention with the Suicide "Attempter"

Many persons who are successful at committing suicide may actually have been crying out for help and were not really intent on killing themselves, but their suicide plan was too effective. Some may have been manipulators who were playing a dangerous and deadly game of scaring loved ones into giving in to their demands. Others had made the conscious and voluntary decision to end their lives and therefore were only waiting for the "right" time.

If, however, someone is able to intervene with a suicide "attempter", there are steps that can be taken to help prevent the suicide. The intervention strategies used with an adolescent suicide "attempter" are similar to those used for adults. Your intervention suggests to the "attempter" that his or her life is of value because someone is interested in saving it. By intervening you allow the individual to release some of the tension causing his or her feelings of hopelessness, and you also provide support to a psychologically weak person.

You can help to prevent someone from committing suicide by talking to the person about his or her suicidal thoughts. It is a myth that if you talk about suicide to a potential victim it will drive him or her to do it. While talking, try and assess the lethality of the person's thoughts. Determine:

- If he or she has a specific plan and method and access to the means.
- If there is a history of prior suicide attempts or if anyone in the family has committed suicide. Also, find out if the person has experienced any other type of significant loss.
- If he or she has recently taken alcohol, tranquilizers or other forms of drugs.
- If he or she is involved in any meaningful relationships and/or lives alone.
- If he or she is depressed and has a marked absence of plans for the future.

Listen to the person and validate his or her feelings. Do not trivialize, reject or deny the person's feelings. Instead get him or her to externalize, for example, feelings of hostility.

If you are in a crisis situation where the suicide is imminent, try and buy time. The longer a potential suicide victim takes to decide, the higher the chances that the person will not take his or her life. You can use this time to help him or her to arrive at alternate solutions to his or her problem. You can also talk about the funeral and the consequences of the person's death on the lives of loved ones. You can emphasize the fact that the depressed feeling will pass, that death is irreversible, and that as long as there is life there is hope.

In addition to talking to someone who is threatening suicide, you should inform others, a family member or someone who is in a position to monitor the person's behaviour and who can do something about the threat. Act specifically to try and relieve the stress felt by a person at-risk. For example, make a phone call to a counsellor or put the person in touch with a suicide prevention centre or hospital.

All suicide attempts must be taken seriously. It is better to risk being manipulated than to have the guilt of someone's death on your conscience. If a person has a history of repeated attempts, however, then this person should be referred for psychiatric help. You may also need to inform the person that you are unwilling to allow yourself to be imprisoned by his or her behaviour any longer.

Intervention with Surviving Family Members
Family members of a person who has committed suicide are not only left with a sense of loss but commonly also experience feelings of shame, fear, anger, rejection and guilt. Many persons believe that of all the different types of bereavement loss, the loss of a loved one by suicide is the most difficult to bear.

Obtaining the services of a counsellor can prove helpful for family members because often no one (within the family or circle of friends) wants to talk about the death or listen to family members speak of it. Therefore, a counsellor can fill the existing communication gap by being available to speak with survivors. Intervention should begin as soon as possible after the death, before family members have a chance to create a distorted picture of what happened. The bereaved can be helped to realize and identify their varied feelings. For example, shame is felt because of the social stigma that is attached to taking one's life; anger arises because of the feeling of rejection; guilt occurs because family members feel responsible for the death or feel that they could have done something to prevent it; fear exists because survivors speculate that suicide may also be their own fate; and a sense of abandonment is experienced because survivors interpret the victim's actions as deliberate and the loss as sudden and without preparation.

Surviving family members may need help to explore and test the reality of their feelings. Much of the guilty feelings may be unrealistic and, with counselling, they can find relief. There are times, however, when there is culpability and in such situations the survivors will need help to cope with their valid feelings and not allow the guilt to consume their being.

There may also be the tendency for suicide survivors (like bereaved adolescents in general) to either idealize the lost one as being super mom, dad, child or spouse, or create an unrelenting negative picture of the victim. Negative or positive fantasizing can result in their having difficulty later on forming or maintaining intimate relationships. Family members therefore should be helped to retain accurate perceptions of the deceased.

In addition to these suggestions, the reader can find other intervention strategies for working with the bereaved in the final chapter of this book.

CHAPTER 7

Death by Murder and from AIDS

Are there Losses that Require Special Attention?

It is no longer uncommon in many societies to have cared for someone whose life was snuffed out by a murderer or by the disease AIDS. I have had a friend die of AIDS in New York at the age of 28 and an uncle who was gunned down by thieves on the streets of Kingston in 1994. Their deaths were, and still are, frightening, dramatic and traumatic, and coping with the losses did not seem to fit into the typical or traditional models for understanding grief.

Death by Murder

There is much commentary on how desensitized some societies have become to murders, due to the frequency of its report in the news and the violence of crimes portrayed in movies, as well as the violent lyrics used in many pop songs. When a murder becomes not just another statistic, but happens to someone with whom we are familiar, however, we find ourselves reexamining issues of mortality and morality. A murder provides us with proof that at any moment and without warning we, or someone we care about, can be deprived of life. Our beliefs about right and wrong and the meaning and purpose of life are shaken. We are forced to face the unpleasant realization that good people are not necessarily rewarded in a manner that we would like.

Few researchers have noted the effects of murder on family members and how this loss differs from a nonviolent one. Sprang and McNeil (1995) have suggested that the bereaved who mourn a loss by murder can feel like victims, as they may never be able to successfully explain the reason for the death. There is usually an excessive concern or preoccupation with the degree of brutality or suffering associated with the crime and an inability to prevent the event from consuming their lives.

The feelings of numbness that a bereaved person typically experiences upon initially hearing news of a loss seem to be magnified in the person who is confronting a death by murder. Denial of the loss can also be prolonged. As with any sudden deaths, because family members are deprived of saying goodbye, there is a tendency to deny the loss. In addition, with murder, the family is sometimes prohibited from viewing the body of the victim because of the state of the body; a decision that sometimes seems to facilitate denial. As has been cited elsewhere in this book, grief counsellors feel that viewing a body in repose seems to help families grieve.

The bereaved family also tends to have strong feelings of rage and hopelessness. The rage can be directed at the suspect(s) or convicted criminal(s) involved in the case and/or the criminal justice system. If loved ones do not perceive justice to be served then they are deprived of a target for this anger. I remember a young lady telling me, some months after her brother was killed, that she had been insanely angry for months with everyone and everything. She described the anger as "eating her out" and it was not until she made a decision to let the negative thoughts and anger go that she was able to reclaim her life. The apparently slow-turning wheels of the criminal justice system can maintain this rage. Families may find that the long drawn out police investigations and court hearings keep them focused on the crime. Thus, they are not able to begin resolving their loss until after the murder trial.

Some persons who are attempting to cope with a loss by murder have been found to acquire new behavioural responses which supposedly serve to "protect" them. For example, they may purchase weapons and security systems or they may restrict their social activities, for instance by refusing to go out after dark. Some may also engage in what appears to be phobic-avoidance reactions, such as performing elaborate actions to avoid seeing the crime scene or any stimuli related to the trauma.

Another effect on family members can be observed in their interpersonal relationships. The bereaved can socially isolate themselves because of their grief as well as because of society's reaction to the death. In order for society to feel safe in a world that seems to have gone berserk, some of its members may psychologically distance themselves from the relatives of a murder victim. I have heard persons recreate a crime in order to reassure themselves that the murder would not happen in their family. For example, people will attribute the death to carelessness of personal safety by the victim or to a motive related to the lifestyle of the deceased, or his or her occupation. Such rationalizations can create a rift between bereaved family members and those in their social circle.

Intervention

A primary goal, immediately after the news of a death, is to help family members stabilize their emotional, physical and social situations. Whoever is with them can help to do this by being supportive and not challenging the defenses raised by the bereaved. Their feelings should be validated, their reactions normalized and their physical needs and comfort addressed.

Attempts should be made to help the bereaved regulate their physiological symptoms of arousal. Up to days after the news of a death the body may go into a continuous state of arousal, where it is difficult to sleep and the person feels "on the alert", prepared for fight or flight. During this stage the bereaved can be helped to become aware of the connection between their thoughts and emotional responses. They can also be encouraged to comfort and nurture themselves so as to reestablish some sense of internal control.

Family members should be closely monitored for critical indicators of suicidal or homicidal ideation. This may arise from the strong feelings of hopelessness, anger or self blame that can accompany this loss. Gradually, the bereaved can be educated about what to expect emotionally and practically over the long and short term. When it is felt they are emotionally ready to do so, the bereaved can be encouraged to say goodbye to their loved one. They should also be helped to integrate the meaning of the experience into their life script so as to feel some mastery over the trauma.

Death from AIDS

Another death that has been found to produce shock waves in its wake is by the acquired immune deficiency syndrome (AIDS). AIDS is a viral syndrome which depletes the body's immune system of its ability to defend itself against life threatening illness. The Division of Disease Prevention and Control of the Pan American Health Organization/World Health Organization (PAHO/WHO) reported 362,004 AIDS-related deaths over a ten-year period to December 1996 in the USA. In Jamaica the records from the Epidemiology Unit, Ministry of Health, indicate 1,320 deaths reported from 1983 to September 1997.

When someone has AIDS, he or she is judged socially and morally, for many reasons. Despite facts to the contrary, there is the perception that AIDS exists only among stigmatized groups, such as homosexuals, intravenous drug users and heterosexuals who have multiple sexual partners. In addition, the infectivity of this disease and the fact that it is found primarily among youths can cause panic and prejudicial behaviour (Moss 1991).

Grieving the loss of a loved one from AIDS shares some commonalities with loss by suicide. Both share the characteristics of being stigmatized grief. In both, the bereaved are forced to grieve in silence because of misunderstanding associated with the loss. At times the bereaved may feel unable to claim their right to fully grieve the loss of a recognized relationship, because the cause of death is not perceived as being sanctioned by society. Family members may therefore lose the usual social support afforded in bereavement.

When the cause of death is stigmatized, it is also often the case that the deceased gets blamed for his or her death. This can create a double-bind situation for the bereaved relatives. On one hand they may find themselves wanting to disassociate themselves from their loved one who has died; at the same time there is the need to stand by and somehow "protect" the reputation of the deceased.

Of all losses, grieving a stigmatized loss especially exemplifies how the bereavement experience is not an individual or isolated event. The impact is experienced by members of the entire nuclear family, as well as the extended family and significant others. We find that with stigmatized grief a large number of persons may be experiencing feelings akin to disenfranchisement.

The often secret survivors of an AIDS-related death commonly report feelings of shame, guilt, abandonment, anger and rejection (Mofatt 1986; Maharajh and Sakar-Crooks 1995; Sprang and McNeil 1995). Other cognitive and affective responses include confusion, panic attacks and denial. Denial is dominant because of the nature of the disease. There is usually a period at the beginning of the illness, after the person has been diagnosed as having contracted the human immunodeficiency virus (HIV positive), when he or she shows no observable physical changes. If family members are informed at this stage they tend to be disbelieving, denying the illness, and have high hopes which prevent them from realistically preparing themselves. Thus, although there exists time for anticipatory grief work, it has not been commonly utilized by this population.

In the majority of cases, family members are informed near the end of the illness. This does not allow them time for "anticipatory work". It may also be that, even if persons were informed early, the stigma associated with the disease prevents meaningful preparatory grief work during that time. Denial is often then continued after the death, primarily because of the existing social stigma.

Anger is another reaction that tends to be prominent among those mourning an AIDS-related death. The bereaved find themselves angry at God for "allowing" the loss to occur. Sprang and McNeil (1995) note that this is especially so when the person has acquired AIDS through a blood transfusion. God is seen as allowing the relative to have the medical condition that necessitated the transfusion. Anger at God, however, may be difficult for the bereaved to vent because of the guilt involved and the religious taboo. Therefore, it is usually displaced onto mortals.

The medical community can be at the receiving end of displaced anger. Family members can perceive them as being insensitive to the patient's needs or as being ineffective. Coworkers, friends and even strangers are sometimes targets for anger. Additionally, anger can be directed at the deceased for acting or making decisions that caused their own death, or the bereaved can be angry at themselves for somehow not preventing the tragedy.

As a result of these angry feelings, the behaviour of the bereaved tends to be affected. Some may show uncharacteristic aggressive behaviours, while some engage in avoidance behaviours. There have also been reports of increases in the incidence of suicide and substance abuse among this population.

Intervention
As is the case with helping the relatives of patients with any terminal disease, intervention involves facilitating communication among all involved by helping persons deal with

their feelings and images about the illness and death. Also, both the AIDS patient and family members can be helped to set new goals for their lives.

After the death, bereaved family members may feel that they have no one to speak to regarding their loss. Persons who are in "helping roles", therefore, should be prepared to listen. There are unique themes of secrecy, protection and control that arise from an AIDS-related death. These need to be addressed with family members so as to minimize the additional stress associated with this type of death.

Counsellors should not be afraid to touch family members. They should act in a manner that encourages the bereaved family to trust them. Those who have worked with this population have found that trust does not come easily, possibly because of the reaction of society to the disease and the ways in which it is contracted.

The reader is referred to other suggestions and information in chapter eight, which can also be used as a guide to intervention in losses that require special attention.

CHAPTER 8

Intervention

How Can I Help Others with Their Grief?

In a review of the literature for evidence of effectiveness of bereavement counselling, Murray Parkes (1980) found that, although everyone did not need professional help, those who did and who received assistance showed a reduction in their psychiatric and psychosomatic symptoms. The relatives of terminally ill patients in a continuing care unit in Aberdeen who participated in a research project showed similar results (Pottinger 1991). Those relatives who received professional support and assistance from the staff prior to the loss reported better adjustment than those who had not received any help.

Another study I conducted at a hospice in Kingston indicated that there are mediating factors such as age that can heighten or lessen the potential benefits received from counselling (Pottinger and Alexander 1990). At this hospice, of those who received prebereavement intervention from the staff, the elderly caregivers of hospice patients experienced less shock and distress at the loss compared to young caregivers who received intervention. On a whole, regardless of intervention, the older caregivers as a group were less distressed than their younger counterparts; a finding that has been supported in the literature (Ball 1977). Age therefore seems to intervene in the impact of loss. It may be that younger persons are not as prepared or experienced in coping with death and thus are at risk for poor adjustment.

Murray Parkes (1980) also found that counselling was most beneficial to those who did not perceive their families as being supportive. Many bereavement experts have concluded that the unavailability or inaccessibility of emotional support for the bereaved places them at special risk for a complicated adjustment. In addition to age and the presence or absence of a social support network, other "at risk" factors that have been well researched with conclusive findings include the history of previous losses experienced by the bereaved person and the relationship he or she shared with the deceased.

It has been suggested that past losses and separation do have an impact on current losses (Worden 1982). Those persons who have experienced previous losses (including losses not related to a death) can either be better prepared to manage a current loss or may feel overwhelmed by another loss. The outcome seems related to how bereaved persons have coped with previous losses. If they experienced a complicated grief reaction in the past, they will likely find it difficult to cope with the present loss. Murray Parkes (1986) has suggested that persons who have a history of depressive illness are at risk for poor adjustment. Also, there is some evidence that loss of a parent in childhood predisposes one to poor coping skills and psychiatric problems (Jacobson and Ryder 1969).

The type of relationship one shared with the deceased is crucial in determining the impact of loss. Pathological grief reactions have been most commonly associated with relationships that were characterized by dependency or ambivalence (Murray Parkes and Weiss 1983). Persons who share a highly dependent relationship probably have poor self-images to begin with. Losing the "strong one" in that type of relationship can devastate the already weakened ego and create exaggerated feelings of helplessness and desperation. On the other hand, the "strong one" who gained his or her strength from the dependent relationship can experience extreme feelings of powerlessness, insecurity and abandonment at the loss.

Worden (1982) believes that an ambivalent relationship is the type of relationship that most frequently results in complicated grief. In highly ambivalent relationships, the survivors are usually left with excessive feelings of anger and guilt because the relationship they shared with the deceased was characterized by conflicts and a mixture of love-hate feelings. Therefore, relationships that are dominated either by ambivalent feelings or dependency do seem to complicate the grief response in survivors. Murray Parkes and Weiss (1983) have proposed that ambivalence creates difficulties for persons in emotionally accepting the loss, and dependency interferes with the ability of survivors to develop new goals and move forward.

The aim of intervention with the bereaved is to help them resolve their loss so that they can carry on meaningful relationships and lead productive lives. Resolving a loss does not mean that grieving is finished forever. Certain aspects of the lost relationship will always remain with the bereaved and there will be times, long after the death, when they will experience pangs of grief. When someone has resolved a loss, either by him- or herself or with assistance, this means that the individual has actively addressed the meaning and impact of the loss and has integrated the loss appropriately into the rest of his or her life.

Intervention with Children

It is difficult for children to work through their grief without guidance. This intervention can be provided by parents, teachers, adult friends, and if necessary professional counsellors. There are certain qualities that a good "intervener" needs. He or she needs to be a good observer who communicates to the child feelings of sensitivity, warmth, acceptance, and a desire to understand the child. The "intervener" needs to be able to allow the child to ventilate his or her feelings, even if the feelings are intense. Also, the child should be allowed to describe his or her own concerns, rather than the "intervener" trying to diagnose the child and unintentionally dictating the child's needs.

Communication with the bereaved child needs to be simple and direct. Using euphemisms such as "Mummy is gone to sleep forever" may be interpreted literally by the child. The aim is to get the child to accept the finality of the loss. Attitude is important when communicating with the child. In fact the child will probably "hear" your attitude more clearly than your words. The intervener's tone and voice therefore should reflect his or her feelings. In addition, adults need to express their feelings around children so that they can receive the information that it is okay for them to express theirs.

As a rule, children tend to mirror the feelings of adults. Thus, young children who have difficulty with their grief are likely to have parents who are not coping well with their loss. A mother once brought her three-year-old daughter to see me. She described the child as having regressed in her behaviour since the death of her father six months previously. Her daughter, who had been potty trained, had begun wetting her bed and clinging anxiously to her. When I attempted to speak to the mother about how she was handling her husband's death, she refused to accept that she would benefit from talking about her response, although she admitted to marked changes in her affect and behaviour.

The person attempting to help with a bereaved child should try to maintain an open relationship with the child, so that he or she feels free to approach the adult at any time. Even when children understand what you have already told them, they may repeatedly ask the same questions. This is not done to annoy you but the child may be seeking reassurance or confirmation of what you have said. By repeating your responses you may be helping the child to actualize the loss.

In addition to helping the child to process the loss as factual and irreversible, the role of the "intervener" is also to help prepare the child about what to expect. The child can be told what to expect of his or her grief reactions, what to expect at the funeral, and also of the practical consequences of the loss. The "intervener" should also use the opportunity to reassure the child that although there will be changes in his or her life, he or she will continue to be taken care of and loved.

Intervention with Adults

Teresa Rando believes that the first step the bereaved need to take to resolve the loss is to give themselves permission to feel and grieve in their own way. She has defined grieving as allowing yourself to "feel feelings, think thoughts, lament loss and protest pain" (Rando 1988). Emotions and thoughts that may be upsetting, unacceptable or uncharacteristic of the individual's normal response style need to be confronted and laid to rest.

When resolving a loss the bereaved also need to make a conscious decision to take each day as it comes and plan to continue interacting with the living. Although there may be a strong urge not to communicate with others, the bereaved need to learn to accept social support over isolation. This will help to promote their emotional health. In addition, the bereaved should work on maintaining good physical health through a proper diet, sufficient sleep and regular exercise.

Although it is not necessary, there are times when the bereaved may need to carry out a ritual to signify the end of grieving or the beginning of their life without the deceased. One young man planted a tree to symbolize he had forgiven his brother for committing suicide. On the first anniversary of their three year old son's death, his parents released helium balloons into the air. Special dates such as the anniversary of the death, birthdays and holidays are significant occasions on which to perform "goodbye rituals".

It was Shakespeare who said "Give sorrow words, the grief that does not speak knits up the o'er wrought breast and bids it break" *(Macbeth* IV, III, 208). Professional intervention is based on this premise. It is healthy for the bereaved to express their grief. There are two options facing the bereaved who feel they need professional help to work through their grief. They can either be referred for counselling on an individual basis or referred to a self-help group where the bereaved meet and support and counsel each other.

The aim of therapy can be to provide insight to the bereaved or offer support. Individuals who have difficulty resolving their loss because of interpersonal and intrapsychic conflicts will benefit from insight-oriented psychotherapy. This form of therapy identifies the existing conflicts that are preventing effective grieving, of which the bereaved are not aware. Over a number of sessions the therapist attempts to show the bereaved client the association between his or her present behaviours and the conflicts. When insight is achieved this usually results in the disappearance of the maladaptive behaviours or symptoms. If the dysfunction involves a family, then a family therapy approach is considered.

Supportive psychotherapy is indicated when the bereaved have insight into their behaviours but need help in reducing their anxiety, strengthening their defenses, and generally restoring their former equilibrium. Most concerned persons can offer supportive therapy; however, a trained person who can access the deeper levels of consciousness of a bereaved person is necessary for insight therapy.

Self-help groups, the alternative to individual therapy, are run by bereaved persons and at times can be supported by a professional. The groups are therapeutic because they offer support, encouragement, guidance and role models to their members. In addition, the bereaved will receive accurate information and practical suggestions at these groups. Such groups help persons to regain their self-confidence and to find purpose and meaning to their lives through the opportunity to help others. Although some bereaved people end up using the group as a crutch that allows them to keep mourning, many derive long term benefits from the group and move on with their lives.

Termination of therapy, in any form, requires planning and forethought. This is an important stage in the therapeutic process because the bereaved is being asked to say goodbye to someone on whom he or she has come to rely. The therapist's aim is not to reawaken feelings of loss in the bereaved. Thus, the bereaved person should be informed well in advance of the final session. This is especially necessary in the case of individuals whose grief response is complicated.

At times I have found that clients will pick a fight with the therapist just prior to termination because it is easier for persons to "let go" of someone with whom they are angry. At the time of termination, which should be mutually agreed upon by therapist and client, the therapist could inform the client of his or her availability for future contact.

Those who are interested in professional help are likely to be concerned with (1) how to find appropriate help and (2) when to seek the services of a professional. Counselling or referral services for the bereaved can be obtained at hospices or other terminal care centres attached to hospitals, at university counselling centres, the local chapters of Cancer Societies, bereavement support groups for any type of death and groups with loss-specific concerns such as for AIDS, cancer, suicide survivors, or miscarriages. Counselling may be obtained at churches, community health centres, from funeral directors and also private practitioners in mental health. Some counsellors at these sources may have little or no training and experience with the bereaved. Therefore, it is the responsibility of the person seeking help to locate the services of a specialist or someone who is sufficiently knowledgeable about the field.

When is professional intervention necessary? If the bereaved think they need help, or if close relatives or friends suggest that they should get help, or if a professional refers them for counselling, then these are considered valid indicators.

If the bereaved speak of the deceased in the present tense and act as if the deceased is still with them, and if they have relinquished their ties to family and friends, then these behaviours warrant intervention.

Any bereaved person who has expressed suicidal thoughts or displayed addictive behaviours should seek help, especially if they are isolated and have no family or friends.

Finally, professional intervention should be sought if the bereaved have suddenly developed physical or psychiatric symptoms, or if they behave in ways that repeatedly cause them to be rejected, lose self-esteem or experience unnecessary loss.

Intervention should not be restricted to only after a loss has been experienced. Research findings suggest that help can be effectively offered to those who are anticipating a loss, such as the relatives of terminally ill patients (Kane et al. 1985; Pottinger and Alexander 1990). The time before a death can be used to take care of matters that should be heeded before the loved one dies. If the hurts are attended to and forgiven this may mitigate the feelings of guilt and distress following the loss.

I am in no doubt that grief counselling or intervention does work. In addition to evidence presented by researchers such as Vachon et al. (1980), Worden (1982), Murray Parkes (1986) and Rando (1988), I have seen marked behavioural changes in the bereaved who have received help. Recently, a young lady entered counselling, approximately eight months after both her parents had died. She was grossly underweight, severely depressed, and unable to perform simple tasks. After four sessions she had started gaining weight, appeared alert and responsive, was able to resume her work and could once again travel on public transportation.

After grief counselling, the bereaved usually report feeling relief from pre-counselling symptoms. Some of these symptoms abate abruptly once insight is achieved, while others fade more gradually with the strengthening of the ego. William Worden (1982) has suggested that there are three types of changes the bereaved experience that can help one to evaluate the results of therapy:

(1) The bereaved should report subjectively that they are feeling different.
(2) They should show observable behavioural changes.
(3) There should be clear and measurable signs indicating that the symptoms have been relieved.

Many persons, after going through a grief experience, with or without professional intervention, discover an inner strength with which to face new challenges. Their view of what is and is not important for happiness changes and their life takes on new meaning and purpose. Some say that the loss has taught them to be more independent and to pursue their goals. Some turn to soul searching and aspire to be better neighbours. Some seek new challenges and make major life changes. And for some, who have been both humbled and empowered by the experience, the prayer by Reinhold Niebuhr becomes their creed:

> God grant me the serenity to accept the things I cannot change
> Courage to change the things I can
> And wisdom to know the difference.

APPENDIX

Final Remarks

What can the bereaved teach us? The thoughts and feelings they have shared with me have helped me to compile this book. After reading it you should be able to answer the following questions:

- What is grief like?
- When faced with loss what are our options?
- Why does grief have to be so painful?
- Is it different for children?
- Why didn't she say goodbye?
- Are there losses that require special attention?
- How can we help others with their grief?

My work with the bereaved thus far has generally shown that those who have suffered losses have much to teach us. But maybe those lessons will be better learnt if we hear them from the bereaved. An interview with a bereaved mother is presented, in almost its entirety, to help us gain more insight into the grief experience, so that maybe we will become better counsellors, friends, relatives or coworkers to the bereaved. (To protect the privacy of the individuals, no names have been used; the interview is recorded here with the consent of the participants.)

Interviewer: And how old was (she) when she died?

Mrs T: She was five years, three months.

Interviewer: So it's almost three years now . . .

Mrs T: May coming will be three years.

Interviewer: I'm going to ask you now to just talk about how it happened.

Mrs T: (Sigh) It just happened . . . (pause) The Friday evening we picked her up at school she was quite happy . . . went to the supermarket together. As usual she would rush first to the bookshelf. She picked up her book and said she would take this one and said "Mommy buy this for me." So we have this game now (mother's face is lit with a smile as she recalls) where I would sneak the book and let her father pay for it . . . on Saturday I wake up and I went to the hairdresser. (She) was with my niece and her sister. When I was leaving she said, "Mommy I'm not feeling well." I said, "What's happening to you?" She said, "I don't want any breakfast." I said, "Okay," so I gave her an orange. When I went back home, they said she was sleeping. So I went in to check on her and she was sleeping normally. Then when she wake in the evening, she came up to me and touch me and said "Mommy I want to pee [urinate]." I lift her up to take her to the bathroom and realized she was having a high fever. So I called my girlfriend at the pharmacy and asked her to send some medication for me. Later we had this function at church and she was feeling better when she woke up, so I said, "Okay, let's go to church." When I was at church, I noticed she was restless. Then I started giving her fluids because I didn't know if she could get dehydrated or something. Then she just started getting into convulsions, shaking and shaking and everybody was asking what is this? Myself and her father were scared and we rushed home. After the convulsions, when she came out, her fingers and body were hooked up, drawn and thing (mother demonstrated) and we called another pastor and called my girlfriend at the University Hospital and she said to rush her over. In the car, she just went unconscious. It was the first we were experiencing anything like this. When we reached the hospital, the nurse felt her and said, "Well she's warm, let's rush her into casualty." Then they took her from my arms and put her on the stretcher. A whole lot of mucus came spewing out of her mouth at that point then. The doctor and nurses looked at me and said, "Oh Mrs T, she's dead."

Interviewer: Oh dear, that was it?

Mrs T: So I was saying "Why? Why? Why?" Because when you look at her she was just a healthy child, looking like she's sleeping. I got so angry. I felt so angry. So the doctors and everybody started to hold me because they figured I was going to explode. So I said "No! Just, just leave me alone!" And the nurse said, "Mrs T, there's nothing we can do." I felt so mad. It's like, God why are you allowing this to happen? And then I reflect back to some years ago when a pastor once said that when he read in the Bible where it says "In all things you must give thanks." He did not know what it meant until he looked at his mother in the casket and he remembered to say thank you Lord and it just came forcibly to me – remembering that.

Interviewer: At the hospital.

Mrs T: Yes, and I looked at her and said out loud, "God is this what it means in the Bible when you say 'in all things give thanks'?" One mind of me was saying well this is one time I'm not going to give thanks. And then another mind was saying, you have to give thanks. So I said, "It's hard but I thank you anyway," and I felt different, completely different.

Interviewer: Right there and then

Mrs T: It's like the strength that I needed just automatically came. But it was still hard. After I said that I say all right I'm fine and I was rubbing her because she was fat and everything. The doctors were looking as if they were saying this is strange. Then they said they can't keep the body because they pronounced her dead there and said we would have to report it at the police station. So I sat back in the car with her in my lap . . . I didn't feel any fear. I didn't feel anything.

Interviewer: Was it a numb feeling, like you were in shock?

Mrs T: No it wasn't that. I just felt like okay she has been with me and she's gone and if this is what it take to do my last for her to the end, I am going to do it. I felt that strength, because when you look at people, everybody was kind of scared and I said, no somebody is going to have to be strong. Because my pastor wife, she was like freaked out, my husband was spaced out. While I sat with her in my lap, I was just reflecting on all the happy times. I've never remembered her being sad. If I just beat her, like she do something, she come back and she hug me and say "Mommy I'm sorry." We were just happy. So I was there reflecting on all these things . . . when I put her on the stretcher (at the funeral home) I bend down and said to her, "Okay, bye. Mummy will see you later." My husband got so upset then, that's when he walked away across the street and he break down (mother started crying at this point). Then he came back and said, "Come, let's get out of here." We drove home and we cried and cried . . . (pause) but that wasn't the cry that I wanted to come out. And then the hardest part was when we got to her grandmother and she asked, "Did they admit her?" That was the hardest part, when I said, "No, she's dead." I just drop on the ground and I cried. Then I hold on to (my big daughter) and cried (pause). After a while I say to myself look at (my daughter). If she sees you like this it can tear her apart. So I said no, because everybody was crying. I said if God gave me the strength at the time when it happened, somebody has to pull us all out of this. So I said to everybody (she) is gone but that does not mean life stop . . . and her grandmother said "Why this have to happen?" And I said "One thing I know nothing don't really happen unless God allows it to happen." And it was, it was so hard.

Interviewer: Did the doctors say what happened, what was the cause.

Mrs T: Okay, (she) is out of school for the least little cold she gets, so (her doctor) said, "Mrs T, you have to be very careful with her because her lungs are in such a bad condition that they can collapse at any time. And I was like okay. But because my whole family have a lung problem I didn't take it serious. And she (the doctor) showed me how to give oxygen if she's getting an attack of asthma. But she didn't have a cold and when she had the convulsions, there was no way I could think that . . . so I don't know. I still don't understand. Because the autopsy said bronchial pneumonia, but some doctors say they think it was a viral infection that attacked the brain.

But from how she came out of the convulsion and she was hooked up and hands clawed, I remember praying and saying to God, for my healthy looking child that I have if this is what you're going to give me back, I don't want her. I definitely prayed that. So what I used to console myself after is like probably I prayed and God answered me. Because that convulsion that she had it's like it had affected the brain and I would get a vegetable and I could not deal with her being a vegetable. The thing that really shocked teachers and everybody is that she was too brilliant, she was just too brilliant. At age five, she completed grade two and they were in a problem what can they do with a child this advanced. They cannot put her with the ten-year-olds. I didn't know what to do, because everything she would read. She would pick up the *Gleaner*, anything. There was no argument that she could not participate in. She was just too advanced for her age.

Interviewer: When you were talking about the sequence of events a while back, was the memory as vivid as three years ago?

Mrs T: I saw everything. It was like (pause) at the funeral it pained my heart to see the little children. They were looking so sad and thing and I felt scared. I don't know where this force came from but I got up, I had to say something. So I said to the children, "Don't you go about and thinking that God is bad to take (her) away from you. He is not bad. I mean some of us have five years, some ten, and some ninety-nine years. It's just that her time is here and she is gone, but the fact remains that God is still good."

Interviewer: Let me ask, do you think of her everyday?

Mrs T: I do. People keep saying, you know, don't talk about her. I just can't understand why people do that because memories don't die. No matter how you try, you cannot blank them out. So as far as I'm concerned, I am driving on the street and I see little children and I will say (she) will be that big now, or she will be doing this. When I hear children doing things, I will say, like, how come when she was that age, she never behaved like them?

Interviewer: So she lives on in you?

Mrs T: She lives on. The thing about it, people will come to the house and say "why is that family picture still there?" I said but that's a part of my family. I don't see why I should abandon her. It's like (someone I know) who lives abroad, he don't mention her. It hurt me. Because of that, the closeness that we used to have, we don't have it. And like the children are scared so I say don't come back.

Interviewer: Some people are just very uncomfortable. They're afraid that if they bring it up it may . . .

Mrs T: Look, if everybody was like me. When you lose somebody, you lose the person, the body, but the memory is still there. Don't make sense you hide and block it out. I remember at one stage I was dwelling on the negative side. Everyday I keep remembering how I saw her dead and the bad parts were overpowering the positive. And I remember one morning I woke up and said, "Lord this thing just have to stop. This evil part of this grieving thing, it's like haunting me. I'm asking you, just take this grieving out of my system."

Interviewer: About how long after the death you remember saying that?

Mrs T: After the funeral, for two weeks people keep coming around, and after that, about one month after, when you're alone, when everybody gone out of the house, in the morning, it was like a depression coming on me. I'm driving on the road and I felt tears coming in my eyes. It was getting to me. I remember as if something was saying "How come you were so strong during everything, now you're just a weakling?" Things like that. I said okay, okay, well I guess this must be a part of it.

Interviewer: It is.

Mrs T: I just have to go through it. I am going through it and I just have to deal with it. And it's like that was about a month after and I remember praying. When I look back that is the time I think that people should change their way of dealing with people who are grieving. Don't leave them alone at that time.

Interviewer: The month after?

Mrs T: The month after, people are there for the funeral and they are there with you a week after. But that's not the time when you need them. It's the month, two months, three months after. Friends stop calling, relatives don't know how to talk to you. And people avoid you. That's not what you need. You need for people to say, "How are you coping? You dealing with it?" Don't act as if you have a disease that you must stay there and deal with by yourself.

Interviewer: I see . . .

Mrs T: And I think this is when most people hurt. Because there are times when you need to talk to somebody. That was a time for the family when it drew us closer because you had nobody else to relate to. And you just barely going through, barely, because nobody is around.

Interviewer: Mmm . . . mmm . . . alright. Yes. Let me just stick with that point a bit. Was there anytime when the relatives and friends were all around, that you felt it was too much company or you always welcomed the company?

Mrs T: No. When everyone was around that was the hardest part and it was not only me it affected, but it affected (my daughter) as well. She felt sick and tired of seeing all the people and wished that they could leave her alone. The part I can't see about it is that even though people say we're supposed to do it because you are supposed to be happy when someone has died – the eating and the drinking . . . I am here grieving, I am mad and to me they are so happy with the merrymaking.

Interviewer: Mmm . . . mmm . . . I have heard a number of people say the same thing.

Mrs T: I just can't deal with it. The more people come around is the more you have to go over the same thing, and right during that time it is just tearing you down. It is doing worse to you.

Interviewer: Alright. Looking back now, was there any particular person or event that helped you to cope, to move on?

Mrs T: Well, my pastor abroad, one of them. He was the person who baptized me and I usually call him my Dad. He called and said "Listen, I know you are strong. I know you from you were a child. I know you have it within you." And just those words . . . I know that helped. And then I know definitely with all that is going on, if I did not have this belief that I have in God, that he is the strength behind everything, I couldn't cope. Because when people come up and say, "What, you daughter dead? Me would have to go down in the grave with her." These things don't do me anything, they don't help . . . I remember someone called and said, "What is this I'm hearing?" I mean I could not believe the nerve of the woman speaking to me in the tone of voice. I said to her, "What you talking about?" She said, "That you kill off my baby." I wanted to just slam the phone down . . .

Interviewer: A lot of people just don't know what to say or how to say things at these times.

Mrs T: As long as I live, I'll never let that woman call back my house. Because she is going to tell me about killing off my child. If there is ever anyone who is dedicated to their children. There is nobody like me. Which other woman would give up all so that you can be there to pick your child up, to help them with homework, to carry them to music. I mean I could be there getting on with my life but I had to be there. I mean I'm against grandmas looking after children, I am against helpers. I did all this, all this sacrifice so I can be there for them. I mean really that thing got to me.

Interviewer: What about the first anniversary of her death. How was that? Was there any particular thing that happened that stands out in your memory?

Mrs T: Well I don't know if I was scared about it or what. But just the thought of it coming up to the time. Believe me even though for the whole of that year I was strong, deep within I was and I know I am still grieving. It affected everybody, because my husband he internalized it, he got sick. I went through a lot throughout that year. I decided to work, just work, just work, to try and keep it out. Because what happen is when I'm alone I just keep on thinking. You know depression is evil. It just let you think why this happen to me etc. So I find that when I'm up and about and meeting with people I feel different. During that year I lost my car as well. I remember saying, is this going to end, and then I just got sick. The day of the anniversary, I woke up and just could not move and when I went to the doctor I was having pneumonia. I am wondering was it really there or just thinking that this is what killed her. I don't know, but it was pneumonia.

Interviewer: I'm going to move on to how has her death changed your life if in any way at all?

Mrs T: I have learnt to appreciate people more. I don't take people or anything for granted anymore. And what it has done for me is made me realize that life is not just life, but death is a part of life. I wish everybody could understand that. I am here for today, I don't know about tomorrow. So okay, I am going to do the best I can for today. What I can do, I am going to live today like it's the last day that I have, you understand? I learn to appreciate everything.

Interviewer: Would you use the word "strengthened" in describing how the loss has affected you?

Mrs T: Yes. I have been, because all my life I am the smallest in the family so I always have people taking care of me. I got married young, so my husband was there to take care of me. And then when she died, that was when my inner strength had to come out because I had to take care of everybody. So it has really strengthened me.

Interviewer: Well you have shared a lot. I am really grateful for this. I am going to wrap up now. Is there anything else you want to share with bereaved persons or persons who have to comfort the bereaved?

Mrs T: I think what I have been doing is saying to people who going through it, look I'm not going to be a hypocrite and say this is easy. It is hard but tell yourself, if it wasn't you, it would be somebody else. And we all have to go through it. Just as how we wake up and we see today and we have to go through it because you are still alive, you just go through it . . . and I tell myself that I am going to go through it with all the energy that I have . . . (pause) and you know what, when people say things like I know how you feel, they don't. And when they say why don't you get pregnant again? Why don't you replace her? I mean how can you replace somebody. It's not a piece of paper that blow out in the breeze. So you just say, that's not me. Leave that alone, I'm not replacing her because I cannot replace her. You know, probably I do it sometimes and annoy them, but people must just leave you. If you want to cry, leave you and let you cry, scream if you want. Be by yourself if you want to. Give you some privacy. But sometimes people impose on you and they keep on telling you, you need to, you need to. Boy, I think you should leave the person. Ask how you think you will be comfortable. Just be comfortable. As far as I'm concerned, I know some mothers may try and drag their daughter (the surviving one) out and say you have to do this. But I say, is that the way you are comfortable. I did that and I notice that eventually she (her other daughter) is coping with it.

Also what I think we need here is support groups. We have support groups for so many things, drugs, AIDS, etc. But we need them for people who have lost someone, especially a child, a young child. I think that's the worst type.

Interviewer: Well thank you so very much, Mrs T. I found this very helpful and I am sure the readers will benefit from the insights and experiences you have shared. Thank you. Thank you.

As was illustrated in the interview, trying to say or do the "right" things when comforting a friend, coworker, or family member can lead to social blunders. Many of us, after such an encounter, are left wondering, did we say or do the "right" thing? A British researcher, Gorer (1965) wrote: "Nowhere is the absence of an accepted social ritual more noticeable than in the first contacts between a mourner and his neighbours, acquaintances or work mates after bereavement" (p. 57).

Anyone who has been in the position of offering comfort understands what Gorer meant. Bereaved persons can be intensely sensitive and often they perceive remarks or gestures offered in condolence as unhelpful, or even insulting.

Presented below are ten examples of attitudes or expressions which bereaved persons commonly perceive as unhelpful:

❖ Telling someone who has recently lost a loved one that "God knows best" may not be perceived as comforting at that time. The recently bereaved are usually angry and have a need to blame and God sometimes gets blamed for "taking" the loved one. Even if they cannot accept the loss, for it to be suggested that they must appreciate it can be perceived as insensitive.

❖ Attempting to console by telling a grieving person that he or she is "holding up well" can be construed to mean that the bereaved should not grieve because they are "strong" when they do not. This expression can force the griever to hold in feelings and pretend, so as not to "let down" their consoler.

❖ Another unhelpful condolence can be to remind a bereaved parent that he or she is young and therefore can have another child; or to tell someone who has lost a spouse they can remarry. The bereaved person may be able to appreciate that fact at a later date; however, during their moments of grief they want back the lost one, not another. In addition, what may be perceived as being suggested is that the deceased person can be easily replaced.

❖ Sometimes in comforting the bereaved we bring up our own experience with loss. The timing of this is critical. If the bereaved person wants to talk about his or her loss and you are interjecting with your own experience, this may not be helpful. The bereaved person may want to feel that his or her grief is unique because the person was so special to them. On the other hand, if the need is indicated, it can be comforting for the bereaved to realize that they too will get over the loss, because others have.

❖ Many bereaved persons have commented that they experience anger when someone says to them, "I know how you feel". This condolence seems to leave the bereaved feeling that you are trivializing their loss. If you have not experienced a loss yourself and you wish to sympathize, it may be more helpful to say "I don't know what you're going through, I can only try and imagine it."

❖ Women who have had miscarriages or stillbirths are sometimes not allowed sufficient time by their friends and family members to grieve. It is a common misperception that these women, as well as expectant fathers, will easily resolve their loss because they never had quality time to bond with the deceased child. Because of this misperception, these bereaved persons may feel that they are not to grieve.

❖ A similar misconception by those in comforting roles is that they should encourage a mother to become pregnant shortly after the loss of a young child. This has been found to be unhelpful if the mother has not yet "accepted" the loss of her deceased child. Such a parent will not likely be in a position to reinvest emotions in a new relationship with another child and subsequently accept this child as having his or her own personality.

❖ Grieving is considered timeless by experts in the field, but often we will either verbally or nonverbally communicate to the bereaved that "it is time to move on". This can put pressure on the bereaved to stop mourning for a loved one because of the expectations of the consoler.

❖ Encouraging the recently bereaved person to move house, relocate or migrate shortly after the loss has generally been found to be unhelpful. This is so because the bereaved person tends to lose the support of family and friends and the feeling of security, stability and predictability with such a move.

❖ Many persons believe that crying is a necessary release for the bereaved. However, this seems to be more a cultural need than biological. Thus, to encourage or force someone to cry may not be helpful, as this can create additional stress on the bereaved to respond in a certain way. Crying is not the only expression of grief. One can grieve without tears. Therefore, what should be encouraged is the expression of grief in a manner in which the bereaved person feels comfortable and which is socially acceptable.

It is hoped that the above suggestions have not resulted in further confusing the reader as to how to respond to the grieving person. My advice generally is to take your cues from the bereaved. A simple expression of sympathy or an acknowledgement of your helplessness may be preferred to a flowery statement of condolence. As a Caribbean person, I believe that one should not withhold expressing sympathy out of fear of intruding on the private grief of the bereaved. However, this should not be seen as a universal practice, as I found out through personal experience in Aberdeen!

My research into death and dying has been a learning experience about living. I have been taught that loving and being loved are not our birthright. Before we can give or receive love in a healthy relationship, we have to learn how to first accept and love ourselves. We have to learn that each one of us has the power to make his or her life happy. Also, love has to be worked at and when we are willing to invest in love, we are placing ourselves at risk of being hurt. But loving is fulfilling and we cannot afford to restrict our growth by harbouring fears of loss and rejection. I truly believe that the experience of loving and living, even though it may be short lived, is worth the inevitable separation. And the pain and hurt that may seem permanent at the time are truly not.

Over the years I have collected a number of "sayings" and poems about loss. These, I have found, have helped me to express thoughts of solace and comfort and to communicate understanding of a feeling or experience. I end this book by leaving a sample with you.

****

The loss of a loved one is one of the most intensely painful experiences any human being can suffer, and not only is it painful to experience, but also painful to witness, if only because we're so impotent to help.

(Bowlby 1980, p. 7)

****

They must go free like fishes in the sea, or starlings in the skies, whilst you remain on the shore where casually they come again

(Frances Cornford)

****

Will this unteach us to complain?
Or make one mourner weep the less?
And thou – who tell'st me to forget,
Thy looks are wan, thine eyes are wet.
(Lord Byron, "Oh! Snatch'd Away in Beauty's Bloom")

****

Whenever Richard Cory went down town
We people on the pavement looked at him:
He was a gentleman from sole to crown,
Clean favored, and imperially slim

And he was always quietly arrayed,
And he was human when he talked;
But still he fluttered pulses when he said,
'Good-morning' and he glittered when he walked.

And he was rich – yes, richer than a king,
And admirably schooled in every grace:
In fine, we thought he was everything
To make us wish that we were in his place.

So on we worked, and waited for the light,
And went without meat, and cursed the bread
And Richard Cory one calm summer night
Went home and put a bullet through his head.
    (Edwin Arlington Robinson, "Richard Cory")

****

Death ends a life but not relationships, which struggle on in the survivor's mind toward some resolution which they may never find.
    (Robert Anderson, "I Never Sang for my Father")

****

. . . Then slowly the world came back: or I myself returned, but to another world.
    (Introduction to the *Collected Poems of D.H. Lawrence*,
      written after the death of his mother)

****

Just as broken bones may end up stronger when healed, so the experience of grieving can strengthen and bring maturity to those who have previously been protected from misfortune.
    (Murray Parkes 1986, p. 5)

****

If I can endure for this minute
Whatever is happening to me,
No matter how heavy my heart is
Or how 'dark' the moment may be –
If I can but keep on believing
What I know in my heart to be true,
That darkness will fade with the morning
And that this will pass away, too –
Then nothing can ever disturb me
Or fill me with uncertain fear
For as sure as night brings the dawning
My morning is bound to appear.
(Helen Steiner Rice, "This Too Will Pass Away")

****

. . . We are troubled on every side, yet not distressed; we are perplexed, but not in despair . . .

For which cause we faint not; but though our outward man perish, yet the inward man is renewed day by day.

(II Corinthians 4: 8, 18)

BIBLIOGRAPHY

Anderson, Robert. 1988. *The Cambridge Guide to World Theatre*, edited by Martin Banham. Cambridge: Cambridge Univ. Press.

Ball, J.F. 1977. "Widow's grief: the impact of age and mode of death", *Omega* 7: 301–33.

Bentovin, A. 1986. "Bereaved children" (editorial), *British Medical Journal* 292: 1482.

Binger, C.M., A.R. Ablin, R.C. Feurerstein, et al. 1969. "Childhood leukemia: emotional impact on patient and family", *New England Journal of Medicine* 280: 414–18.

Bowlby, J. 1969. *Attachment and Loss: Vol. I. Attachment.* New York: Basic Books.

Bowlby, J. 1980. *Attachment and Loss: Vol. III. Loss, Sadness, Depression.* New York: Basic Books.

Byron, George Gordon. 1945. *The Poetical Works of Lord Byron.* London: Oxford Univ. Press.

Cornford, Frances. 1954. *Collected Poems.* London: Cresser Press.

Elkind, D. 1984. *All Grown Up and No Place to Go.* Reading, MA: Addison-Wesley.

Engel, G. 1961. "Is grief a disease?". *Psychosomatic Medicine* 23: 18–22.

Figueroa, J.P., A. Brathwaite, E. Ward, et al. 1995. "The HIV/AIDS epidemic in Jamaica", *Current Science* 9: 761–68.

Folkman, S., R. Lazarus, C. Dunkel Schetter, et al. 1986. "Dynamics of a stressful encounter: cognitive appraisal, coping and encounter outcomes", *Journal of Personality and Social Psychology* 50: 992–1003.

Garland, A., and E. Zigler. 1993. "Adolescent suicide prevention: current research and social policy implications", *American Psychologist* 48: 169–82.

Greene, M. 1993. "Chronic exposure to violence and poverty: Interventions that work for youth", *Crime and Delinquency* 39: 106–24.

Gorer, G. 1965. *Death, Grief and Mourning in Contemporary Britain*. London: Cresset Press.

Jacobson, G., and R. Ryder. 1969. "Parental loss and some characteristics of the early marriage relationship", *American Journal of Orthopsychiatry* 39: 779–87.

Jenkins, C.D. 1971. "Psychological and social precursors of coronary disease", *New England Journal of Medicine* 284: 307–17.

Kane, R., S. Bernstein, R. Rotherberg, et al. 1985. "Hospice role in alleviating the emotional stress of terminal patients and their families", *Medical Care* 23: 189–97.

Kaprio, J., M. Koskenvico, and H. Rita. 1987. "Mortality after bereavement: A prospective study of 95,647 widowed persons", *American Journal of Public Health* 77: 283–87.

Kastenbaum, R. 1985. "Death and bereavement in later life". In *Death and Bereavement* I, edited by A.H. Kutscher. Illinois: C.C. Thomas.

Kastenbaum, R., and R. Aisenberg. 1976. *The Psychology of Death*, concise ed. New York: Springer Publishing.

Kubler-Ross, E. 1969. *On Death and Dying*. New York: Macmillan.

Lawrence, David Herbert. 1928. Introduction to *Completed Book of Poems*. New York: Penguin Books.

Maharajh, H., and P. Sakar-Crooks. 1995. "A feeling for revenge", *AIDS Window* 6 1: 4–5.

Moffatt, B. 1986. *When Someone you Love Has AIDS*. New York: Nal Penguin.

Moss, V. 1991. "Patient characteristics, presentation and problems encountered in advanced AIDS in a hospice setting – a review", *Palliative Medicine* 5: 112–16.

Papalia, D., and S. Olds. 1992. *Human Development*, 5th ed. New York: McGraw-Hill.

Parkes, C.M. 1965. "Bereavement and mental illness. II. A classification of bereavement reactions", *British Journal of Medical Psychology* 38: 13–26.

Parkes, C.M. 1970. "'Seeking' and 'finding' a lost object. Evidence from recent studies of the reactions to bereavement", *Social Science and Medicine* 4: 187–201.

Parkes, C.M. 1972. "Components of the reaction to loss of limb, spouse or home", *Journal of Psychosomatic Research* 16: 343–49.

Parkes, C.M. 1974. *Bereavement Studies of Grief in Adult Life*. London: Tavistock Publications.

Parkes, C.M. 1980. "Bereavement counselling: does it work?", *British Medical Journal* 281: 3–6.

Parkes, C.M. 1986. *Bereavement Studies of Grief in Adult Life*, 2nd ed. London: Tavistock Publications.

Parkes, C.M., and R. Weiss. 1983. *Recovery from Bereavement*. New York: Basic Books.

Pigou, E. 1987. "A note on Afro-Jamaicans' beliefs and rituals", *Jamaica Journal* 20: 23–26.

Pine, V. 1989. "Death, loss and disenfranchised grief". In *Disenfranchised Grief: Recognizing Hidden Sorrow*, edited by K. Doka, 12–23 Toronto: Lexington.

Pottinger, A.M. 1990. "The role of expressing feelings before bereavement: a cross-national study of relatives of cancer patients in Aberdeen and Jamaica". PhD dissertation, University of Aberdeen.

Pottinger, A.M. 1991. "Grieving relatives' perception of their needs and health in a continuing care unit". *Palliative Medicine* 5: 117–21.

Pottinger, A.M., and D.A. Alexander. 1990. "Do relatives of terminally ill patients also benefit from hospice care?", *West Indian Medical Journal* 39: 239–42.

Rando, T. 1984. *Grief, Dying and Death. Clinical Intervention for Caregivers*. Illinois: Research Press.

Rando, T. 1988. *Grieving: How to Go on Living When Someone You Love Dies*. Lexington, MA: D.C. Heath.

Raphael, B. 1977. "Preventive intervention with the recently bereaved", *Archives of General Psychiatry* 34: 1450–54.

Raphael, B. 1984. *The Anatomy of Bereavement: A Handbook for the Caring Professions*. London: Hutchinson.

Rees, M., and S. Lutkins. 1967. "Mortality of bereavement", *British Medical Journal* 4: 13–16.

Rice, Helen Steiner. 1972. *Someone Cares – The Collected Poems of Helen Steiner Rice*. New Jersey: Fleming H. Rennell Co.

Robinson, Edwin Arlington. 1950. "Richard Cory". In *The Oxford Book of American Verse*. New York: Oxford Univ. Press.

Sanders, C. 1989. *Grief, the Mourning After: Dealing with Adult Bereavement.* New York: John Wiley & Sons.

Seligman, M.E.P. 1972. "Learned helplessness", *Annual Review of Medicine* 23: 407–12.

Selye, H.L. 1976. *The Stress of Life*, 2nd ed. New York: McGraw-Hill.

Sprang, G., and J. McNeil. 1995. *The Many Faces of Bereavement – Nature and Treatment of Natural, Traumatic and Stigmatized Grief.* New York: Brunner/Mazel.

Stroebe, M., and W. Stroebe. 1987. *Bereavement and Health: The Psychological and Physical Consequences of Partner Loss.* New York: Cambridge Univ. Press.

Thielman, S., and F. Melges. 1986. "Julia Rush Diary: coping with loss in the early nineteenth century", *American Journal of Psychiatry* 143: 1144–48.

Vachon, M.L.S., W.A.L. Lyall, J. Rogers, et al. 1980. "A controlled study of self-help intervention for widows", *American Journal of Psychiatry* 137: 1380–84.

Walsh, F., and M. McGoldrich (eds). 1991. *Living Beyond Loss: Death in the Family.* New York: W.W. Norton.

Worden, W. 1982. *Grief Counselling and Grief Therapy.* London: Tavistock Publications.

Yodder, L. 1986. "The funeral meal: A significant funerary ritual", *Journal of Religion and Health* 25: 149–60.

INDEX

Abnormal grief. *See* Pathological grief
Acceptance: of loss 8
Adolescents, grief response in 33-34;
Adolescent suicide 39-43; case studies 41; and stress 42; and the availability of firearms 42; Garland and Zigler on 40-41, increase in 41; reasons for 42
AIDS: and social stigma 51-52; coping with death from xvi, in Jamaica xvi, 51; death by 47; grief response to loss by 51; intervention for loss by 53-54; in the USA 51
Anger, in adolescents 34; as grief response 5, 6; response to murder 48-49

Ball: on age factor in grief response 56
Bentovin: on behavioral changes in bereaved children 33, 34
Bereaved: mortality rate among 26; and new relationships 19
Bereavement: and suicide 37-45; as loss xiv-xv; in children 31-36
Bereavement intervention. *See* Grief counselling
Bereavement overload 25
Bereavement research. *See* Grief research
Bereavement response. *See* Grief response
Bereavement rituals 60. *See also* Christian rituals, Death rituals, Irish wake, Jewish rituals
Binger: on response to sibling death 35
Blame: as grief response 6; religious–philosophical perspective 27
Bowlby, John: on depression among bereaved 23-24

Children: and bereavement 31-36; and divorce 12; intervention for bereaved 58-59; and loss 32; and parental loss 34; parental response to bereaved children 35; preparation for bereavement 36; response to grief xv; sibling death 35
Christianity: and death 29-30
Chronic grief. *See* Pathological grief
Complicated grief. *See* Pathological grief
Confusion: as grief response 3
Crying: as grief response 5
Cultural perspective: and the bereaved 20; and death rituals 28

Death from AIDS. *See* AIDS
Death: and Christian philosophy 29-30; by violence 31
Death by murder. *See* Murder
Death rituals 27-28; and Irish wake 27; and nine-night 28; Christian 29; Jewish 28

Delayed mourning, 16-17; in unresolved grief 16
Denial: as grief response 1-2; in response to loss through AIDS 52
Depression: as grief response 23; and suicide 39
Divorce: and relationships 13; as loss 11-13

Elkind, D: on stress in adolescents 42
Emotional support, in the bereaved 17-18
Ethno-focal theory 20, 21, personal vs social beliefs 22; Pottinger on 22
Expression of grief 17-18; influence of health professionals 22; Pine on family influence on 22; significance for healthy adjustment 59-60

Firearms: role in adolescent suicide 42
Folkman, S. et. al: on stress research 26
Funerals, as turning point in grief 4

Garland, A. and E. Zigler: on adolescent suicide 40; on warning signals of suicide 38
Gorer, G: on changing traditions and bereavement 29
Greene, M.: on crime in the USA 31
Grief. *See also* Pathological grief, cultural perspective 20-21; acceptance of 4, 8; bereavement overload 25; confusion in 3; denial in 1-2; intervention strategies xvii, 58-61; phases 1, 3, 7, 8
Grief counselling xiii-xiv, 55-56; insight therapy in 61; to effect grief resolution 61; intervention for coping with suicide 45-46; supportive therapy in 61; termination of 62

Grief expression. *See* Expression of grief
Grief research xvii; case study 66-75
Grief resolution 7, 8, 17, 57, 59-60;; and age 55; and depressive illness 56; and intervention with children 58-59; closure in 60; role of support groups 2, 17, 60, 61; significance of counselling for 61
Grief response 3, 5 16; age factor in 56; in children xv, 31-36; depression, 23; to multiple loss 16-17, 56; to loss by murder 48; withdrawal 24; religious–philosophical perspective 27; *See also* Delayed mourning, Masked mourning
Guilt; as grief response 7: and suicide 45

Health professionals: influence on grief expression 22

Irish wake 28
Insight therapy. *See* Grief counselling

Jacobsen, G. and R. Ryder: on persons at risk for poor loss adjustment 56-57
Jamaican death rituals 28
Jenkins, C.D.: on mortality among the bereaved 26
Jewish death rituals 28

Kaprio, J.M. et al: on mortality among the bereaved 26
Kastenbaum, R.: on bereavement overload 25
Kastenbaum, R. and R. Aisenberg: on modern society and adolescent suicide 42
Kubler-Ross, E.: on loss 1

Learned helplessness 25
Loss adjustment. *See* Grief resolution
Loss: acceptance of 4, 8; and attachment 23-24; from AIDS 51-53; children and 32; effect on surviving family members 18; feelings of 8; by murder 48-49; and multiple loss 16-17, 56; of parent in childhood 56; of spouse 25; processing of 3-4, 7; psychological effects of 10; reactions to 5; relationships and 13; types of xiv-xv, 1 *See also* Bereavement

Maharaj, H. and P. Sakar-Crook: on grief response to stigmatized loss 52
Masked grief: as unresolved grief 16; psychosomatic reactions 16
Modern society: and adolescent suicide 42; murder in 47
Moffat, B.: on grief response to stigmatized loss 52
Mortality: and the bereaved 26
Moss, V.: on AIDS and social stigma 51
Murder: behavioral response to 48-49; coping with death by xvi; and the desensitizing of modern society 47-49; intervention for coping with loss by 50; psychological response of bereaved to 50; societal response to 49
Murray Parkes, Colin: on children and bereavement 34; on coping and religion 27; on counselling as bereavement intervention 56; on grief resolution 56, 57; on grief response 8; on loss 1, 8

Nine-night: Jamaican death rituals 28
Nolan, Nikola: case study on grief response in divorce 11-12

Parental loss: effect on children 34
Parents: response to bereaved children 35
Pathological grief 15-16; effects of ambivalence on loss adjustment 57
Personal belief system: and response to death 21
Pigou, E.: on Jamaican death rituals 28
Pine, V.: family influence on grief expression 22
Psychological autopsy: profile of suicide victims 39
Psychological effects: of bereavement 10
Psychosomatic response: to grief 4,6
Physiological response 3-4; to murder 50; to stress 26
Pottinger, A.: on counselling as bereavement intervention 55; on hospice care 55; on the ethno-focal theory 22; on stress of bereavement 27
Pottinger, A.M. and D.A. Alexander: on socioeconomic status and grief 25

Rando, T.: on intervention for bereaved 59-60; on preparing children for bereavement 32
Raphael, B.: on loss 1
Rees, M and S. Lutkins: on suicide among the aged 15
Religious–philosophical perspective 27-30. *See also* Christianity, religious rituals, death rituals; as coping strategy, 27
Religious rituals: and death 28
Relationships: and divorce 13; and grief 10, 57; forming new 19

Rituals. *See* bereavement rituals, Christian rituals, Irish rituals, Jewish rituals, religious rituals

Sanders, C.: on response to sibling death 35
Self-help groups: role in loss adjustment 61
Selye, H.I.: on physiological response to stress 26
Separation anxiety 24
Shame: and suicide 45
Shock: as grief response 1-2
Sociocultural perspective. *See* Cultural perspective
Sprang, G. and J. McNeil: on anger in response to loss through AIDS 53; on effects of murder on family members 48; on grief response to stigmatized loss 52
Stigma: and AIDS 51, 52; effect on grief response 52; and suicide 40, 45
Stress: and adolescent suicide 42; and grief 25, physiological response to 26
Stroebe, M. and W. Stroebe: on stress and depression 25
Suicide: and adolescents 39-43; and the aged 14-15; and depression 39; and guilt 45; and surviving family members 45; as grief response 14, and shame 45; intervention strategies 43-45; persons at risk for 37-38, 39, 44; psychological state of victim 40; reasons for 40; social stigma 40, 45; statistics in the USA 14,15
Support: in grief resolution 17, 18; the need for 2

Therapy. *See* Grief counselling, Self-help groups
Thielman, S. and F. Melges: on the religious-philosophical perspective in bereavement 27

Withdrawal: as grief response 24
Worden, W.: on children and loss 33; on effects of previous loss 56; on forming new relationships 18-19

Yodder, L.: on Jewish death rituals 28

www.ingramcontent.com/pod-product-compliance
Lightning Source LLC
Chambersburg PA
CBHW071233170426
43191CB00032B/1511